Weight Loss:
How to Keep Your Commitment

Jonni Good

Wet Cat eBooks

Wet Cat eBooks.
For information please write:
4820 SW Greensboro Way #46, Beaverton, OR 97007
jonni@howtothinkthin.com

ISBN 0-9741065-0-X

Printed in USA

For Jessie, of course.

ii

Thanks

I want to take this opportunity to thank some of the many people who offered the support and advice that I needed in order to bring this project to completion.

First, I want to thank Christine Macgenn Rodgerson. Christine is the author of the inspirational *A One-Legged Cricket*, and has written many books and articles about alternative medicine. I am extremely grateful that she took time out from her busy schedule to offer her invaluable suggestions and support. This book would never have been written without her encouragement at every step of the way.

I also want to thank Faith Haugen for reading my very first rough draft. She's been cheering for me from the beginning.

And I especially want to thank all the readers of my *How to Think Thin* email newsletter. I've never met these folks in person, so I'm always surprised when so many readers take the trouble to let me know that my efforts are making a difference — one life at a time. And that's what it's all about, isn't it?

iv

Contents

Congratulations!

You've just made a decision that could change your life. Weight Loss: How to Keep Your Commitment gives you a specific program that will help you kick the habits that make you fat.

If you combine this book with a healthy diet, you will be able to stay committed to your health for the rest of your life. No more yo-yo dieting, no more failure, no more anxiety about your health.

Naturally, before starting any new diet program, you should talk to your doctor. This book is not a substitute for your physician's professional opinion.

This book is also not a substitute for a true commitment. If you are still "thinking about" losing weight, but are hoping for a way to accomplish it without making major changes in your diet or lifestyle, this book will probably not help you.

If you are committed to repairing your health and getting a thin, beautiful new body, this book will give you the skills you need to give up your addiction to an unhealthy diet full of sugar and fat.

There is a weight loss miracle.

It's called "food." The "secret" to losing weight and regaining your health is to kick the addictions that cause you to eat the wrong food — and then commit yourself to a healthy eating plan that lets you eat all you want and still lose weight.

This book helps you with the first part of that plan — in the next few days you'll learn a system that will allow you to let go of your addiction to sugar and fat.

You should use this book along with a healthy eating plan, so that you will be able to redirect your cravings — you can actually use your sugar cravings to lose weight, if you use the right eating plan. The one I highly recommend to everyone I know is the book by Dr. Joel Fuhrman called *Eat to Live: The Revolutionary Formula for Fast and Sustained Weight Loss.*

This is going to be an exciting time — so let's get started!

Introduction

You want to be able to lose weight and keep it off without the constant, emotionally-draining struggle.

You see people who never seem to eat too much, who always choose non-fattening food, and who stay vibrant and healthy. You want life to be that easy.

Up to this point you may have thought you needed more will power, or that you needed to take the latest "fat-burning" pill, or you needed to eat boring food while obsessing about all the things you really want to eat. You keep fighting your weight problem, and it keeps on winning.

It just doesn't seem fair that some people are able to stay thin without going to all this effort.

It is especially unfair since most thin people have no idea why they make different decisions about food than the rest of us do. They probably believe that they have more will power, more self-control, fewer cravings, and better metabolism. They can't tell you how to think the way they do, because they've never thought any other way — they think its "normal."

For thin people, it is normal. But that doesn't mean that the rest of us can't kick our addictions to unhealthy food and learn to make conscious choices. We just have to learn the process, and practice it long enough to create a new habit of thought. Once we have learned to think differently about our cravings, we can use them to lead us to healthy food that helps us lose weight.

What are the steps you'll take to learn to "think thin" and kick your sugar habit?

First, you'll look at what it is about the human brain that makes you want sugar and fat so much, and how your instincts short-circuit your eating decisions. You'll then be able to replace your self-anger with understanding and compassion — this is the first step towards letting go of the struggle, and taking control of your eating choices.

Once you see how your instinctual mind interacts with your conscious mind, you'll realize that this is the normal way for a brain to work — there's really nothing wrong with the way you think now. It just doesn't work so well in the 21st century, because the foods we naturally crave aren't good for us any more. We misread our natural cravings, and end up addicted to sugar and fat.

Our bodies were designed, whether by evolution or by the Word of God, to live in a world that did not contain white flour, white sugar, refined oils and fats, or grain-fed cattle. Our appetites, which are part of our survival system, are focused toward getting enough of the rare fruits and wild game that existed a million years ago.

Back then, things that tasted sweet were good for us, because ripe fruit is sweet — and full of the nutrients our bodies need. Sugar seems to be good, because it's super–sweet "super-fruit." Our instinctive mind thinks sugar is good for us. It isn't.

Instead, it brings us obesity, diabetes, immune system problems, and other health issues. And it's physically addictive. This is something our instinctive mind cannot understand.

To get more in tune with your real dietary needs, you'll do some fine-tuning so that you will make fully conscious eating choices. You'll then be able to listen to what your body really wants, and eat the food that makes you healthy instead of fat.

To do this, you're going to learn a very simple mental exercise called "walking meditation" that can be used during your commute to work — or whenever you have a few minutes to yourself. This easy and enjoyable skill will help you feel more focused, and more aware of the times when your instinctual mind tries to make eating decisions for you.

Now you'll be able to simply look at the thoughts your instinctual mind uses to convince you to maintain your unhealthy food addictions. You'll look at those thoughts and let them go — without a struggle or internal argument — and make the right choice, the conscious choice, instead. You'll be amazed at how easy this is to do, once you've practiced walking meditation for a very short time.

Then you'll have the chance to look at things in your life that make it more difficult to maintain this state of awareness — and the biggest obstacle for most people is stress.

For that reason, there is a full chapter in the book that shows you how your own thoughts may be adding to your stress level without you realizing it. Ask anyone who is trying to kick an addiction, and they'll tell you that stress is one of the biggest reasons for failure.

To keep stress from sabotaging your weight loss plan, you'll learn exactly how you can use the new skills you've developed in order to reduce that stress level.

By the time you finish the chapter on stress you'll be much more aware of the ways your instinctual mind undermines your weight loss plans, if your addiction to sugar and fat makes you misread your cravings. You'll be making conscious choices about food on a daily basis, which will guarantee your success.

As you continue to practice your new skills, your new awareness will become completely natural to you. You'll see food in a whole new way, and be amazed at how good a healthy diet can make you feel.

Because of your new awareness, you will understand how important it is to create a supportive environment at home and find people and activities that give you the extra support you need. You'll get some suggestions for doing this in the "Practical Stuff" chapters.

And there's a bonus chapter that teaches you an easy meditation — more like a guided daydream, really — that shows you how to give yourself an emotional hug any time you need one. It's about learning to love yourself — something that everyone says you need to do, but no one tells you how. Now you'll know, and it feels great.

By the end of the book you will have a strong program in place for kicking the habits that make you fat. You will also have tools that will free your emotional and mental energy for things in life that are more important than food — because you now trust yourself to make better eating decisions. The internal fight is over.

Because you have that extra mental energy you'll feel more creative and involved in life. You'll be doing things six months from now that you wouldn't even dream of doing now.

In this book I have concentrated on describing only those mental exercises that can be learned quickly, with the least disruption of your daily schedule. If you decide to follow up on any of these techniques and learn more, I have provided a suggested reading list at the end of the book.

And remember — you need to use this book along with a healthy eating plan, like the one in Dr. Fuhrman's book, *Eat to Live: The Revolutionary Formula for Fast and*

Sustained Weight Loss. Dr. Fuhrman has helped thousands of people regain their health and reduce their weight, while eating as much food as they want.

You do have cravings for healthy food — you just misdirect those cravings to unhealthy food because of your addiction to sugar and fat. With Dr. Fuhrman's book, and the skills you are learning now, you can use your own cravings to rebuild your health.

Now, get comfortable, because you are starting on a wonderful adventure — you're going to learn how to change the way you think about food!

How I discovered this program

About seven years ago I finally made the connection between my chronic depression and the almost hypnotically repetitive negative thoughts and memories that constantly filled my mind.

Ironically, everyone I know thinks I'm always in a good mood, simply because I go out of my way to be polite and "nice", no matter what. But inside my brain I was replaying every defeat, reliving every past upset, agonizing over every possible insult.

My brain was a negative mess, and I paid for it with chronic depression. I'm not alone. Millions of people have the same problem. The good news is that as soon as I saw that my negative thoughts were the cause, and not the result, of my depression, I set out to find a way to control those thoughts.

I read through dozens of books by self-help masters, spiritual healers, and modern-day scientific experts who study the workings of the brain. Out of all that information I developed a simple, easy to follow system to change my mind.

It worked. Which was a true miracle, because I had been depressed ever since I could remember.

Did I immediately start to use that same system to rid myself of my excess weight? After all, I'd also been overweight for as long as I could remember.

But no. I didn't make the connection between the way I thought and the way I ate.

A few years later I took the opportunity to go back to college. I chose to take the courses I needed in order to get an addictions counselor's license.

I loved going back to school, doing all the homework, reading all the textbooks. But there seemed to be a lot missing from the regular course of study, so I also dived into the medical journals, on my own time.

I learned that almost all alcoholics and drug addicts kick their habits all by themselves (which is something that very few people seem to know). It's true — most people who become addicted to drugs and alcohol find a way to give them up without going to self-help groups or treatment centers. I wanted to find out how they did it.

It made sense to me — design a treatment program around the same principles and behaviors that work for the greatest number of people. That isn't the way the addictions treatment industry works right now, at least in the United States. But to me, it just makes sense.

I discovered through my outside reading that the mental process that successfully recovering addicts go through is exactly the same process that I went through in order to get free from my chronic depression. The only difference is that most drug and alcohol addicts just naturally find that system because they make the connection between thought and behavior.

It didn't come naturally to me. I struggled to first learn what would work, and then teach myself that system, because it took me forever to make the connection between thought and emotions.

So, now did I use this powerful system to help myself lose my excess weight? No, because I still didn't make the connection between the way I thought and the way I ate.

That took another five years.

There were some very big changes going on during those years, so I did have other things to think about. For instance, I found out I had breast cancer.

I used my new skill in mental control in order to keep the fear of cancer from putting me back into depression.

I knew by then that negative thinking can affect your immune system, so that was my number-one priority. I safeguarded my thoughts the way others would protect their bodies — and I'm convinced it is the biggest reason that I'm now officially a cancer survivor.

It was the five-year mark after my cancer diagnosis that actually moved me to do something about my weight. I needed a way to celebrate that important milestone.

I wanted to give myself a gift that no one else could give me: A thin new body.

Of course, I'd already dieted in the past, like everyone else. And I lost weight on most of those diets. Then, like everyone else, I gained it all back, and more.

I wanted this time to be different.

I honestly don't know what it was that finally made me realize that there was a connection between addictive behavior and my weight problem. Since caffeine is the only drug I've ever been addicted to, maybe that's why it took so long to put two and two together. That "duh" finally filtered into my brain, and I suddenly knew that I had all that I needed in order to lose the extra weight, get healthier, and keep the pounds off for good.

I knew how to change my body, because I already knew how to change my mind.

As simple as it sounds, after seven years I finally woke up to the fact that I was in possession of a secret that millions of people struggle to find — the means of staying committed to a weight loss plan.

My system works. I lost 37 pounds in four months, by replacing the sugar and refined carbohydrates in my diet with real food. I didn't go hungry. I just started to give my body what it is that bodies really need — nutrition.

I still haven't gained any of that weight back, after two full years, and I know I never will. I've broken free of my addictive eating behavior!

When I discovered that others could learn this system and make it work for them too, I put myself on a mission. I was going to get this information out to as many people as possible.

That's why I put together a web page at http:/www.stress-free-weight-loss.com, and why I wrote this book. I want other people to have the freedom that I've experienced by kicking my addiction to sugar and other highly refined carbohydrates, while also taking control of my cravings for fattening junk food.

How is "food addiction" possible?

My behavior around food fit all the hallmarks of classic addiction, and now I know that scientists have proven that the pure chemical substances we love so much — sugar and white flour — are truly addictive.

Here's how to tell if your eating has become an addictive behavior:

- Do you eat foods containing sugar, white flour, or white rice every single day?

- If you were to list five of your "comfort foods" would all of them include refined carbohydrates or butter, olive oil, or some other fat?

- Do you eat for emotional reasons or when you're feeling stressed?

- Does the food you eat to calm down or feel "loved" contain sugar, white flour and fat?

- Do you find yourself "needing" to grab a hamburger or pizza at a fast food joint at least once a week?

- Do you regularly buy French-fries, potato or corn chips, or other deep-fried snack foods?

- Do you feel that "something is missing" if you watch TV without something to snack on?

- If someone suggests that you shouldn't eat any sugar, white flour or fat-drenched fast food, do you instantly reject the idea as absurd?

- Are you feeling slightly uncomfortable just reading this?

- Do you feel a little angry when someone tells you that your diet is unhealthy?

- Are you totally convinced that you can continue to eat sugar, white flour and junk food (but perhaps "cut down a bit"), and still lose your extra weight or improve your health? In spite of the fact that it's never worked in the past?

- When you go without sugar, noodles, bread or other refined carbohydrates, do you feel "strange," slightly woozy, or get a headache or other uncomfortable symptoms?

- When you refrain from eating any candy, bread or other refined carbs, do you begin to obsess about the foods you gave up, or feel "picked on" and grouchy?

- Have you gained more than 10 pounds since you were 20 years old?

- Do you try to avoid having your picture taken?

- Do you avoid looking in mirrors?

- Did you stay away from your high school reunion because you think you're too fat?

- Do you often feel bloated or get indigestion after eating certain foods, but still eat them anyway?

- Do you manage to stay thin (even though you eat sugar and other fattening foods) by spending hours in the gym or because you work at a strenuous job all day?

- When you take a vacation from the gym or work, do you tend to gain weight?

- Do you have any difficulty sleeping, or wake up around 3 a.m.?

- Do you often feel lethargic, moody or depressed?

- Have you memorized the push-button code for your favorite candy bar or snack on the vending machine at work?

- Has your doctor warned you about your blood pressure or told you that you are at risk of getting diabetes if you don't lose weight?

- Do you fully intend to follow your doctor's advice, but just haven't quite gotten around to it?

If you answered "yes" to two or more of those questions, I can easily predict that you have tried at least one diet in the past — and possibly many diets — but always regained the weight. Diet books always tell you that diets don't work. Now you know exactly why they don't work. You're hooked.

Sugar addiction happens the same way that many people become addicted to heroin, alcohol, nicotine and cocaine.

But most Americans get hooked on sugar at a much earlier age.

Almost all addictions have these components:

1. You begin eating, drinking or using something because it feels good or tastes good — or both.

2. You continue because it feels good when you do it, and it feels bad when you don't.

3. You aren't able to stop even though it damages your health, and continue to do it even when the dangers have become obvious.

The only addictions that don't follow this pattern are caused by modern medicine. Pain medication, even over-the-counter headache medication, can cause painful withdrawal symptoms when you give them up. The pills themselves don't make you feel good, but in the beginning they help reduce the pain of your headache.

Because the withdrawal symptoms are very similar to, or even worse than, the pain you first took the pills for, people keep on taking the medication without knowing where the pain is coming from. So, medically-induced addictions leave out the first step (the pleasure). All the other steps are the same.

Recent scientific studies have shown that most people who are hooked on over-the-counter headache medication have no idea that they're physically addicted. When they begin to feel their withdrawal headache (which can be tortuously severe), they reach for the medicine bottle because those little pills make the headache go away.

For exactly the same reason, most people don't know they're addicted to sugar and refined carbohydrates. These "foods" are so common in our society that they appear at almost every meal, and show up at every potluck, celebration, and funeral. The snack machine is full of them; the prepared foods at the supermarket are full of them. Even the "healthy" bran muffins at Starbucks are full of them.

If you're physically addicted to sugar or refined flour, you will go into uncomfortable withdrawal symptoms if you go without these chemicals for even a few hours. And most people assume that the symptoms of withdrawal are actually hunger pangs, or signals that it's time to eat more of these chemicals! And this is one of the biggest reasons why most diets last only a week or two.

Sugar withdrawal symptoms are nowhere near as harsh as the pain that nicotine addicts go through when they stop smoking. And they aren't as dangerous as the withdrawal symptoms that alcoholics experience. But sugar withdrawal symptoms, if you give up all refined carbohydrates, can be uncomfortable for a while.

Yes, there are withdrawal symptoms. And it often isn't easy. But that doesn't mean you can't give up your habit. In fact, compared to many addictions, giving up sugar and other refined carbs like white flour is easy. It's staying "clean" afterwards that's hard.

I recently experienced withdrawal symptoms because I decided to stop drinking coffee. I knew there would be a headache (and there was), so I scheduled my headache for the weekend.

I didn't get much done around the house for those two days, but by Monday morning my headache was gone. Caffeine is addictive, but that doesn't mean I can't stop drinking coffee — it just means I'll pay a small price if I do.

Other drugs, such as tobacco, have far longer and more disturbing withdrawal symptoms. Sugar addiction's withdrawal symptoms, by comparison, are quite mild.

Whether or not you're successful in kicking an addictive habit depends on how you handle three different stages in the process.

The first stage is the status quo — before you've given up your habit. The second stage is the week or two when you experience the withdrawal symptoms that are a natural consequence of removing an addictive substance, like sugar, from your body. The third stage is life after physical addiction — when your habits and cravings still play a part, but when the physical withdrawal symptoms are no longer present.

You'll need to create a desire and a commitment in order to move from the first stage (status quo). It is very important to acknowledge that there are perfectly good reasons why you would like to make no changes — you enjoy the bagel in the morning, you like the taste of sugar, it helps you feel better in the afternoon, you enjoy sharing your baked goods with your friends and family, etc. We all have reasons for eating the way we do now. Acknowledge those reasons — it's an important part of the process.

(At the end of this chapter you'll find the first Action Step that helps you find and nurture a true desire for change. Be sure to do your homework!)

There are also very good reasons for giving up the sugar and white flour habit — it makes you fat, it leads to heart disease and diabetes, etc. You have specific reasons of your own. Get clear in your own mind about what those reasons are.

Look at both sides of the issue, educate yourself as much as possible about nutrition, and then make a specific choice to give up sugar and other refined carbs, or not. If you'd like to learn more about the dangers of sugar and other refined carbohydrates, I highly recommend the book *Eat to Live*, By Dr. Joel Fuhrman.

Once you make the choice to give them up, you are then faced with a few days (or a week or more) with uncomfortable symptoms. This is where many of us fail, in spite of our best intentions. In fact, many people choose not to give up their addictions because all they can see ahead of them is the symptoms they will feel.

With sugar addiction, the withdrawal symptoms may be weakness, slight nausea, headache, and other fairly mild but possibly uncomfortable symptoms. My caffeine withdrawal headache lasted two days, sugar withdrawal symptoms may last for a week or two. Some people may experience little or no discomfort at all.

Instead of seeing a specific beginning and end of those symptoms, they look at it as though there were simply a big red wall. Knowing how long your symptoms will last will give you the strength to commit yourself to moving through the withdrawal stage.

There are many similarities to the process people go through when they give up an abusive relationship. If all you see is the loneliness you'll feel when you leave, without being able to see that the period of mourning will be over in six months to a year, many people never make the first step.

But also, if you don't acknowledge that there will be a period of "withdrawal," you may be tempted to turn around and go back to the one thing you know for sure will make those symptoms go away.

Many people return to abusive relationships, drugs, and bad diets just days or weeks before the symptoms would have gone away on their own.

For this reason, it's important to mark out the time when you know you won't feel your best. Think of it as a voluntary case of the flu, and commit to working your way through it. In a few days it will be over, and you'll be on the other side, looking at a lifetime of health.

Once you've worked your way through the withdrawals, are you home free? No, because cravings for sugar, white flour and fatty foods don't go away. We have a natural, instinctual need for sweet food, and our culture (and yes, our parents) taught us to feed that need with sugar instead of fruit and wholesome vegetables and whole grains.

This natural need for sweet food is so important that we are going to learn, in the next few chapters, exactly how that need came about, and how cravings can actually affect the way you think and behave.

But before you go any further, please do this important Action Step.

Action Step #1

This step is designed for people who know they should lose weight or start an exercise program, but who just can't find the motivation to move them to action. Does that sound like you?

Now I want to make something clear right up front: I can't give you the motivation you need to succeed. But I can show you the steps to take so that you can create your own motivation. We're going to use the proven steps that lead to success, no matter what goal you have in mind.

It's a fact that 95% of dieters fail, and lots of people who sign up for expensive gym memberships never go back to the gym. Why not? It's all in the attitude, as the diet book authors say. But how do you get the winning attitude that creates motivation?

There are three specific steps to take to build that attitude. If you follow these steps carefully, you will be able to truly believe that this time you will be successful, no matter how many times you've failed with your weight loss or fitness goals in the past. It is this personal faith in yourself that will make success possible.

The process I'm going to show you has been used by thousands of people who have become successful in every walk of life. The secrets of success are the same, whether you are reaching for business, health, or spiritual goals. As long as you're willing to follow through on these simple steps, you will create the motivation, the "winning attitude" that you need in order to succeed.

The homework for this first Action Step is going to take some thought. Most people believe they've already done this step, but very few really have.

Here's what I want you to do: Go to a quiet place, or do your thinking on this subject after you've crawled into bed and you turn out the light. You need to have the peace and quiet so nothing competes with your thoughts and the images that you create in your mind.

Now that you are relaxed, think of why you feel a need to lose weight or become more fit. Put this reason in a clearly defined picture in your mind. To do that you'll need to think of a positive reason, not a negative one.

Why? Because "high blood pressure" is hard to turn into a compelling picture. And "Not having pain in my knees when I walk" gets translated in the subconscious mind to "having pain in my knees when I walk."

This assignment is intended to send a very clear message to your subconscious mind, and your subconscious mind cannot understand negatives or abstract thought.

It needs a clear picture of what your life will be like after you've succeeded with your weight loss or fitness goals.

Let's take that example of painful knees and see what we would do with it in order to create a compelling image of success. Many people who carry too much weight have this problem.

Put in your mind an image of yourself walking down a city street, and imagine the feeling of walking in comfort.

Imagine how it feels like to be moving a thinner body. Remember what it feels like now, with your thighs rubbing against each other, and your arms pushed out from your body by excess weight. And then imagine that extra flesh gone. Your arms now swing freely, your legs are moving swiftly, powerfully. You've got a spring in your step.

Be sure to imagine this from "inside yourself" — the image should exactly reflect what it would really be like – (and not you watching a movie of yourself walking down the street). However, do imagine that you catch a glimpse of your reflection in a store window. You're wearing fine clothes on a thin and beautiful body.

If your reason to change is different — perhaps to avoid heart disease or reduce the complications of diabetes — imagine what your life will be like when you've followed your doctor's instructions and your health has improved. Think of the things you now avoid doing, like playing sports or getting down on the floor with your grandchildren, or even building a project for the kids in your back yard.

Then create a clear, believable, and complete picture of yourself enjoying these activities in your healthy new body. Include the sounds, the smells, and the emotions that would accompany this success.

Now you know what it is that you really want, and you've put it in a form that is much more compelling than just saying "I need to lose weight." Write down your image so that you can read it in the morning. Even better, if you have a tape recorder, dictate the words that best describe this image of success. I can't stress enough the importance of this step.

In the morning, after you've had a nice rest, take out that piece of paper or listen to that tape. Repeat the words, and recreate the images in your mind as often throughout the day as you can. You'll be setting the stage for success.

Now read the next few chapters that show you why, and how, your own mind can mistakenly lead you to actions that are not in your own best interest. As you read, and as you go through the next few days, keep thinking about what life will be like when you're free of all your excess weight, and you have become healthier.

Expand on that image, nurture it, and let it grow. As you build on this mental image, be sure to keep writing or recording your thoughts. You'll be making this image much more real for your subconscious mind by following this step.

Use a small notebook and answer the following questions.

- I hope to lose weight because:
- And this will allow me to:
- Which is good because:
- And then I'll be able to:
- Which will mean that I can also:
- Which will lead to:

Instincts and appetites

It isn't your cravings that make you fat — it's what you eat when you feel the cravings. If you're a sugar addict, you've come to associate the cravings with the wrong food, and this misunderstanding leads to obesity and poor health.

All of us enjoy the taste of sweetness, because it's built into our survival system. Some of us enjoy this taste sensation more than other people do, which leads us to become addicted to sugar and other refined carbohydrates.

As we discussed in the previous chapter, we can become officially un-addicted simply by going "cold-turkey" for a week or two — but this doesn't take away our cravings for sugar.

It would be nice if we could simply do away with our desire for sweet food — then it would be so easy to stay on a healthy eating plan. But this is never going to happen.

The reason for this is that the human brain — the part of our brain that does all the thinking, planning, dreaming and creating — is built on top of an old mammalian brain that is in charge of the mundane things, like breathing, keeping the heart beating regularly, keeping the immune system working the way it's supposed to.

Our survival system is located there, in the old brain —which hasn't changed much since we were tiny mammals hiding from the dinosaurs.

Your survival system is in charge of your appetites. If you were a koala bear, you would think eucalyptus leaves taste good. In fact, you'd think they were the only things that taste good. A koala bear's body needs the nutrients in those weird-smelling leaves because his body has evolved for that specific diet.

The human diet is far more varied, but there are still things that we need to eat in order to stay healthy. The most important things for the human diet are fruits and vegetables — specifically ripe fruits and sweet-tasting leaves like lettuce, kale and chard.

For this reason, the desire for sweetness is built in to our survival system, and is never going to go away. It wouldn't be a problem if it weren't for the fact that there is now so much food on our supermarket shelves that appeals to our cravings for sweetness, but which gives us no nutritional value at all.

Mass-produced, highly refined food is abundant, inexpensive, easy to get, and it tastes good. But it doesn't have the same nutrients you find in fruits and wild game.

The problem is not simply that we eat too much — it is the specific things we eat that cause us so much trouble. The biggest enemies of a thin and healthy body are sugar and some kinds of fat — exactly what our cravings lead us to eat, because we have replaced the natural foods with processed, unhealthy food.

Humans aren't the only ones who are willing to eat unhealthy, sugar-laden food instead of the fruits and vegetables we really need. Consider the bear, for instance.

In the wild, a bear will eat berries and fish — and an occasional paw full of wild honey. He naturally eats the things in his environment that his species needs in order to grow and thrive, because his appetites are focused on those foods. His appetites are an important part of his survival instincts.

If you inadvertently offer a wild bear the chocolate cake that you left on top of the picnic table, he'll eat it. In fact, bears love human food, and get just as addicted to junk food as we do. Cakes, cookies, candy and soft drinks are sweet, and the bear's appetites are drawn to them, just like ours are.

Nutritional experts now tell us to eat at least five to eight servings of fruits and vegetables a day for our health. This is a pretty good indication that these foods were necessary for our evolving species a million years ago. Our bodies need the nutrients in fruit. And the sweet ones are the ones that are good for us.

So is it any wonder that our appetite for sugar is so strong?

Because of our natural cravings, if you crave donuts and try to give them up through will power alone, you will feel cheated, deprived, and picked on — so for most of us, staying on a diet is hard. If we had invented manufactured food that tasted like cardboard there would be no problem, would there?

Humans aren't all instinct, of course. We also have a conscious mind that has evolved to allow us to make decisions that are "counter-intuitive." We can actually choose to act in a way that we might not do if we were purely instinctual animals. And we think we're making those conscious choices all the time.

We can choose to eat fruit instead of a donut, even though the donut is sweeter. We can re-train our mind to correctly read our own cravings, and use them to get healthy. This is something our friend the bear would never be able to do.

The biggest obstacle to a healthy diet is something that Alcoholics Anonymous calls "stinking thinking." It's the thoughts that tell us that we need to go back to eating those candy bars and drinking those Cokes.

We convince ourselves that our unhealthy habits aren't really all that bad.

We believe the thoughts that say that we really can lose weight without changing our diet all that much.

We become adamant that the only thing we need is a pill or a special exercise or some other miracle that will let us keep our addiction to sugar and fat, and still get thin and healthy.

These thoughts are a product of our unconscious, instinctive mind, which really believes that we need the super sweet, super fat food we've been eating. In spite of our best intentions, these false ideas can come sneaking into our mind – and if we don't know how to recognize them, we'll believe them! We can actually talk ourselves into doing things we really don't want to do.

Even if you have already given up sugar and fat, and gone through the one to two week withdrawal period, these false thoughts can lead you back into addiction.

In the next chapter, you'll look at what neuroscientists have discovered about the way your unconscious mind works, so you'll have the understanding you need to provide a framework for positive change.

Action Step #2

You may have spent a great number of years believing that you could lose weight, and keep it off, if you just tried harder! I want you to do me a favor. I want you to give up on that idea.

Trying harder is what people do when they choose to follow a plan that doesn't work. Rather than correcting their course, analyzing their successes and defeats in order to create a plan that really works, they do the easy thing. They tell themselves that the original plan has no flaws, contains no lessons, and can't be changed — therefore "trying harder" is the only option that is left.

Trying harder to do something that doesn't work will not bring you success, regardless of your goals.

But allowing yourself to imagine doing something different requires preparing your mind to accept a new idea when it presents itself. If you've held onto a failing plan so long that you cannot allow yourself to give it up, you cannot gain from any new information — possibilities will present themselves to your mind, but you'll be completely unprepared to see them.

That's why we have to do this next step in the process. Two days ago I suggested that you should create a solid image of success — an image that is so real that you can see, feel, and hear it as you bring it into your mind. I suggested that you write this image down, in full detail — or better yet, to tape your own voice as you describe this image of life after you've lost weight and become fit and healthy.

Now, how do you move this image into a plan of action? After all, imagination without action won't help you lose weight.

Therefore, I want you to do this for me. Recall that vivid image of success that you've created. Make your image so real, so vivid, that your new, thin, healthy self can pull up a chair and sit down right beside you.

Now that your image of success is keeping you company, I want you to begin writing down an important list.

How to Keep Your Commitment

The list will consist of all the things you now eat, and all the things you now do, that you already recognize to be unhealthy.

These are things that you enjoy doing, perhaps even love doing, but which keep you from having the body you desire. Be perfectly honest in this exercise — there is no shame in admitting that you enjoy the taste and "rush" you get every morning from your three cans of Coke. If your downfall is watching too much TV, or eating out at fine restaurants famous for their high-fat gourmet food, then write it down.

Search through a typical day and notice every thing that you recognize to be an obstacle to success. Then write it down.

Next, I want you to spend the next two days on this very important project. I want you to keep your image of success very firmly in your mind, and as you think of what life will be like after you've regained your health, look at your list and honestly check off the items on that list that you are willing to give up in order to meet your goals.

I want to make this very clear — we aren't talking about things you're willing to "try" to give up.

As an example, when I wrote my own list two years ago, I saw that "too little exercise" was one of my obstacles. So I sold my car. Even today I still walk 1/4 mile to the commuter train every morning, rain or shine. And every weekend I walk to the grocery store, one mile away. Believe me, there are a whole lot of times when I don't want to. But my car kept me from achieving my fitness goals. So I sold it.

I also saw that my love of baking fine breads and rolls was making me fat. So I threw away all the sugar, flour, baking chocolate and yeast in my house — and gave away my baking pans.

We're talking about burning bridges here, folks. What are you really willing to do to reach your goals?

Everything of value comes at a price. You will soon find out, by comparing your image of success with the list of obstacles, exactly what losing weight or getting fit is worth to you. If you aren't willing to pay for that success by finding a solution to any of the obstacles on your list, then two things are possible:

1. Perhaps you don't value the idea of losing weight or having a stronger body. If this is true, you may as well stop spending money on weight loss books, products and programs, and forget about buying that membership at the gym. You would be far better off if you spent your time, money and creative energy on pursuing a goal that you truly believe to be worth reaching for.

2. Or, you may simply have given too little thought to creating your mental image of success.

Perhaps you included a negative statement that your subconscious mind has misunderstood.

Or maybe you imagine an activity that doesn't really appeal to you — maybe you think it should, because it's something that other people want, but it isn't what you want.

Go back and look at yourself in your strong, thin body, and see yourself doing something that really reflects your own dreams and desires. Work on making that image as emotionally positive as you can, developing it into a completely believable, completely compelling vision.

Then go back and see if you can check off any more of those items on your list of obstacles.

If you find that you are willing to give up a good number of those items, or find a solution to those obstacles, in order to have the body you've built in your imagination, you'll be ready for the next step. You've now looked at what you want out of your weight loss or fitness program. And you know exactly how much your success is worth to you.

Unconscious choices

There isn't anything wrong with your instincts. They are working exactly the way they are supposed to, even when you obsess over the potato chips left in the bottom of the bag. For that reason, you shouldn't get angry at yourself for wanting the chips — but for the sake of your health and your appearance, you need to somehow rise above the craving.

To do that, it helps to know exactly what happens when you make an instinctual choice, so you can recognize when it happens to you.

Of course, humans would like to believe that we are always rational, and that we always make the best decisions possible with the information we have available.

It isn't even close to being true, and neuroscientists have proven it. Our instincts are alive and healthy, and often make our decisions for us. But our brain is built in such a way that our conscious, thinking mind always thinks it's in control.

When I finally realized that I wasn't always making rational decisions, especially when it came to food, things started to make more sense. I had never been able to understand why I could make intelligent decisions about so many things in my life, but still make such stupid choices about food.

Now, maybe you would never do such a thing, but I used to be capable of baking several pans of cinnamon rolls with cream cheese frosting with the full intention of taking both pans to work for a potluck party the next day.

And then I'd eat one entire pan of rolls that night, all by myself.

That isn't rational. It definitely isn't in my best interest. And it wasn't what I intended to do. But I didn't seem to be able to stop. "Something else" took over.

But there wasn't anyone "else" around, so it was obviously me eating all those rolls. I was "of two minds."

And I'm not the only one. If 60% of Americans are dangerously overweight (and we didn't need a scientific study to prove it — just look around at the folks in a crowd), there are a lot of people in our society who do eat more than they should. And even more than they want.

The nutritional experts are right. Instincts still make us crave sugar and fat. Even when we know that sugar, refined flour and most fats are unhealthy, we talk ourselves into eating them anyway.

Alcoholics Anonymous calls it "stinking thinking." Stinking thinking is a great way to think of those thoughts that come into your head and try to talk you into eating just one candy bar, or stop for just one hamburger on the way home from work. You have committed yourself to eat a healthier diet, but part of your brain keeps trying to talk you out of it. And those thoughts can be very difficult to ignore.

But why do these false thoughts sneak into our minds —and why is it so easy to believe them?

Recent scientific studies have discovered that human beings make fewer conscious choices than we think we do. Much of our brain power is actually used to think up excuses for having acted unconsciously. That's why we can do something that we really didn't want to do, and then explain the decision in a way that no one believes but us.

Addictions counselors call it "denial." But we all do it. And there are reasons why this is actually a good thing, most of the time.

Let's look at the times when we are most apt to be making an instinctual, or unconscious, decision.

- When you're doing something that the body naturally associates with survival, like eating.
- When you're in a high-stress situation or in danger.

Scientists have found that when faced with a dangerous situation, humans make a decision about how to react, and actually begin moving, before the conscious mind even knows that anything is happening. Believe me, this is a good thing — you don't want to have to stop and think if you see a giant rock falling straight towards you, or when an enemy soldier is taking aim in your direction.

Our old survival-oriented brain has to have a way to turn off the conscious mind, without our knowing it, so our thinking brain won't get in the way and slow us down when speed is the only thing that will save us.

But this "invisibility" works against us when unconscious decisions are made about matters of diet and health.

As we learned in the last chapter, when it comes to making eating choices in a world filled with manufactured food, our instinctive mind just can't be expected to make healthy, reasonable choices.

Most of the snacks and fast food that are available today were specifically designed to make the most of (should we say "prey upon"?) our instinctual desire for sugar, fat and salt. And we are bombarded with the idea that we need to eat convenience foods because we just don't have time to feed ourselves without corporate help.

Your conscious mind knows that you need more fruits and vegetables, a balanced diet, and more exercise. But when you have an opportunity to make the choice between a healthy meal and a convenient, fattening snack, you often let your instinctive mind make the choice for you — especially when you're under stress. You don't mean to — it just happens.

Then your conscious mind gets the job of thinking up an excuse for it.

Now that you know that this phenomenon happens (not just to you but to everyone), you have the opportunity to learn the simple tricks that have been used for centuries to take conscious control. You can live the life and have the body that you have been wanting for years.

The desire for sweetness can actually work to your benefit, if you deal with it on a conscious, intentional level. That's what you are now going to learn how to do.

So what can you do?

We're going to borrow some simple techniques from the ancient Masters. They call it "living in the present" or "staying awake." Don't worry – you don't need to become a Zen master to learn these techniques. I'm going to show you only those mental exercises that are easy to understand and simple to apply, so that you can begin using them immediately.

And you don't need to change your belief system, because these techniques have been used for centuries by people from all parts of the world, and from all faiths. You will simply be learning how to notice when your instinctual mind is most apt to be taking over your eating choices, and take conscious control. How? Read on.

Action Step #3

You now have two of the three things you need in order to have that "attitude for success."

A few days ago you began to develop a strong, distinctively personal image of what your life will be like after you reach your weight loss and fitness goals.

Then I asked you to keep that image next to you as you wrote down a list of all the things you now enjoy doing and eating, but which are obstacles that stand in the way of your success.

By doing these two things, you should now know if you have a commitment to lose weight, and exactly how much you value that commitment.

Now it's time to move towards action. Remember — desire without action won't create change.

The first step you'll take today will be to create a specific timeframe for reaching your goals. And you'll also write down the exact amount of weight you want to lose, or the specific fitness goals you're reaching for.

If you need to lose weight or get fit for medical reasons, you should also write down the specific items that will prove to you that you have reached your goals. With your doctor's help, find out what your cholesterol counts should be, or what your blood pressure should be.

Also, if you have diabetes or some other illness caused by a poor diet or by being overweight, talk with your doctor to establish a specific goal — perhaps to lower your medication, or reach a specific level of fitness.

You'll be reducing your image of success to numbers on a page, so you can see — on a daily basis — if you're moving towards your goal or away from it. Make the goal specific, like "I will be 40 pounds lighter by Christmas."

How to Keep Your Commitment

Make this as detailed as possible, and keep it where you can easily refer to it. I find that putting my goals on the wall above my bathroom scale is very helpful.

You now have a compelling image of success that you can call on when you need extra motivation. You know exactly how much you value your own personal goal. And you have the specific timeline that you will use to chart your success.

Now all that's left is action.

Now is the time when you should analyze your past successes and defeats with the purpose of learning how to create a winning plan of action.

Remember, keep your mind open so that you don't find yourself "trying harder" to follow a plan that doesn't work. Now that you have built an image of success, and know exactly what that success is worth to you, and now that you have a specific timeline to follow, your mind will be open to the new possibilities that you may have rejected before.

What action you take will depend upon your circumstances and your goals. Without action, nothing happens — but if you have followed the three steps I've outlined, and if you've truly put an honest, solid effort into carrying out the steps, you should now be ready to take the action you need in order to succeed.

You should begin to celebrate every success you experience. That doesn't mean that you should only get excited about the numbers on your scale going down.

It means giving yourself a truly honest pat on the back if you walked a block further than you usually do on the way to work. If you ate a banana or orange on your break instead of your usual candy bar. If you got up an extra half-hour earlier than usual so you could do some aerobic exercises.

Celebrate! Get excited with each successful activity, no matter how small. It is these small skirmishes that eventually win the battle.

By analyzing your failures, I do not mean "feel guilty" when you slip up. I mean that you should look at the circumstances that surrounded that slip, and find a way to change the plan so that it will be less likely to happen again.

If you see that you stayed up too late the night before, you now have a specific choice to make tonight, and tomorrow night. If you feel light-headed or start to slump at a certain time in the morning, you might discover that you need to drink less coffee, or bring fruit so you have something good and sweet on your desk.

Analyze the situation, and then let it go.

If you hold on to a vision of your failures, your subconscious mind will project those same failures into the future. So analyze the problem, create a solution, and then never think about it again. Refocus your mind on your image of success. In the next few chapters, I'll be giving you a specific mental exercise that will allow you to let go of negative thoughts.

This is a powerful skill to learn — don't just assume that "you already do something like that." Do the program! It's the only way to make it work.

Are you getting excited about your future? Are you seeing yourself in your fine new clothes, walking your thin, strong body down the street? Do you now have that motivation, that winning attitude that will propel you to success?

You've now got a vision, you know how much it means to you, and you have a specific plan of action. You're looking towards the future, instead of the past.

Keep these things firmly in your mind, and nothing can stop you from getting the healthy new body you desire.

How to Keep Your Commitment

Walking meditation

Now that you have built and nurtured your commitment for change, you're going to start taking control of your food choices by becoming more conscious of your thoughts. As you learn this technique, you will also let go of the need to pick on yourself for making bad choices, and you will learn how to reduce the amount of stress you bring into your life with angry or unhappy memories.

This new skill will let you kick the sugar addiction that makes you fat — and it will prevent your natural cravings for sugar from leading you back into addiction. All this sounds like a very big assignment, but the steps to freedom are actually easy.

What do you say while you're talking to yourself?

There are some rare and wonderful people who don't think with words, but most of us do. And most of us have words running around in our heads almost all of the time. We call it "thinking."

The first exercise I want you to do is simply to become aware of what you think about, at any given time.

To do that, you'll learn a technique called walking meditation. (If you don't walk all that much, you can also do it in the car on your way to work, although walking is more fun. You can call it "driving meditation" or "riding on the bus meditation" if you want to.)

This may be very different from what you've previously thought of as meditation — especially if you've got an image of sitting in the lotus position (are there really people who can do that?), chanting or staring into a candle. In fact, you can practice this technique while walking down a busy street and no one will even notice.

Be sure to do this exercise, even if you can't see any reason why you should. It is the one essential key to successfully overcoming a sugar addiction, and controlling the cravings. You can't experience it for yourself just by reading about it.

The simple mental exercise called walking meditation.

I want you to simply walk around the block and watch what you think about. You will walk for a few steps, and then become aware that you are thinking about something.

Notice what you're thinking about, and then let it go. Look at the trees, or the cars driving past, and make yourself just see things for a second, without thinking anything.

A few steps later you will notice you're having another thought. Notice that thought too, and let it go.

You'll notice that your mind is almost never empty — and there isn't any reason why it should be. We aren't trying to empty out your brain — just to practice noticing what it is you think about.

You'll discover that you think the most amazing variety of things, because you're not letting yourself stay on any one subject at a time. Perhaps you'll notice yourself thinking that the neighbor's windows need painting around the trim. Remember — notice the thought, and then let it go.

Your next thought may be about the office birthday party that you forgot to buy anything for. You notice, and let it go.

Next you think that this is a silly exercise. You notice, you let go.

You may find that the same thought keeps coming back, over and over. Perhaps you got in a fight with someone at home, and you replay the argument, adding those perfect come-backs that you didn't think of at the time.

That's ok — but remember to let go of it just as soon as you notice yourself thinking about it. And also notice how long it takes you to notice when you are thinking about a highly charged subject, or when you are focused on something that you have often focused on in the past.

And then let it go, and wait for the next thought to pop up. It won't take long.

This can be a rather enjoyable exercise if you lighten up and use a bit of humor. Remember — you aren't trying to change what you think, you're not trying to stop thinking, and you are not judging what you think. Just notice.

Pretty easy so far, right?

Now, begin to take some interest in the environment that you're walking through. Just after noticing a thought and letting it go, turn your mind to seeing the trees and houses or buildings, and feel the sidewalk beneath your feet.

Feel the breeze that is gently playing with your hair, and hear the birds singing in the trees. Then notice that another thought comes into your mind, and that you are no longer focused on the things around you. Gently let the thought go, and once again turn your attention to the world around you.

Keep on noticing, letting go, being aware, and then thinking your thoughts, for as long as you are out on your walk.

You've just practiced walking meditation!

If you have actually done this exercise, you will now be aware of three things:

You can only concentrate fully on one thing at a time.

You can change what you are thinking about, even if only for a few seconds at a time (that will increase as you practice).

You now know what it feels like to "wake up" and live in the present — something that every spiritual master tells us that we have to do in order to take control of our lives.

Taking Control.

Now that you have become more aware of your thoughts and daydreams, you should practice replacing any thought that doesn't bring you closer to the goals of your day. This can actually be any goal, not just about weight loss.

For instance, if you find you are worrying about a conversation you had with your mother on the phone last night, but really need to be putting together a plan for a presentation at work, now is the time to practice taking control of your conscious mind. Gently say to yourself, "No, I would rather think about something else." And then put the new thought into your mind.

If you practice this with thoughts and daydreams that have nothing to do with food, you will give yourself the skills you need the next time you are facing the aisles of the supermarket, or a fattening lunch menu. Thoughts just pop into your mind all the time — but you don't have to keep them there. You can choose what you think about.

When you notice you are making an excuse for wanting to eat something that isn't on your weight loss plan, you don't need to argue with that excuse. Remember, the excuse is just the conscious mind's way of taking credit for a decision it didn't make.

It's perfectly natural, and something that we all do. But the excuse really isn't true — no matter how much we would like to believe it. So we don't have to give it any room in our brain at all. Just see it, and let it go. No internal argument, just conscious choice.

Action Step #4

You've followed the first three Action Steps, which show you how to build and nurture your commitment to health and weight loss. Now the next step (in addition to that all-important walking meditation), is to build up your "will power."

Here's a simple plan that will help you create the persistence and will power that's needed in order to follow through with the decision to lose weight.

Persistence can be nurtured by following this four-step guideline.

1. Discover your true purpose for wanting to go on a diet.

You remember this from Action Step #1. Remember — it doesn't actually take any will power to do something you really want to do. But in order for the subconscious mind to believe you want to do it, it needs a positive image

How to Keep Your Commitment

of the goal you're after. If it keeps hearing you say, "Dang, I have to give up my favorite foods so I can lose weight," your subconscious mind will "help" you get what you really are saying you want — fattening foods.

If you haven't built this positive picture of success, please go back to Action Step #1 and do it now.

Can you truly say you have a burning desire to lose weight? If you can't say that yet, it's a pretty good bet that sooner or later you'll find a piece of chocolate cake on your plate, and you'll have no idea when it was that you gave up on your diet.

So work on this step — nurture it, feed it, build on it —until you feel a compelling desire for change.

2. You need a plan that is reflected in your actions.

Yes, this was Action Step #2. "Intending to" or "trying to" do the plan does not count. Most people stop at this step, simply imagining themselves taking steps towards change, but never actually changing anything.

Don't let that be you. Find the weight loss program that meets your needs, and then act as though it matters each time you make a choice of what you eat. It will matter, if you've paid attention to Action Step #1.

When you get up each morning, think about the choices you made the day before, and compare those choices with the plan you've chosen.

Did you make sure that your plan was reflected in your actions?

If not, recommit yourself each morning. If you find that you never follow the plan, it may be time to reconsider the program, and find one that better fits your needs.

3. Don't allow any negative suggestions to come into your mind from your relatives, friends or acquaintances — or yourself.

They don't mean to, but many people who really care about you will offer the opinion that you've chosen the "wrong program" (no matter which program that may be). They will try to get you to change your mind, in the spirit of helpfulness. Or they'll offer you sweets and treats, saying that "you deserve it, just this once."

Don't allow this kind of loving sabotage to destroy your commitment to health.

And remember that your own internal judge may also offer you negative, discouraging thoughts. Gently move these thoughts out of your mind. If you really desire a thinner, healthier body, you'll need to let go of the habit of picking on yourself.

This is where your walking meditation will truly become your lifeline — it will allow you to say, gently, to your friends and family (and even to yourself!) "Thank you very much, but I've chosen to do this for myself. Please don't try to tempt me or try to change my mind."

4. Join with a group of people who share your burning desire, and who will help you follow through with your plan.

Choose this group wisely. Many people think they're serious about weight loss, but never actually lose weight because they don't really do anything about it. Or, if your friend is totally committed to a program that clearly doesn't work, and insists on encouraging you to follow in her footsteps, she isn't the right person to choose as a "diet buddy."

Look for someone who is already losing weight, and who shows some real excitement about it. She'll love to have your support and encouragement, and her own enthusiasm will be contagious. You can actually gain a lot for your own morale by giving her help when she seems to need it.

But remember; choose your diet buddy wisely. If you don't know anyone who can help you, come join us at the Weight Loss Success Forum at http://www.stress-free-weight-loss.com/forum.htm

We'll be learning more about the importance of support in a later chapter. For now, begin to notice who is really supportive, and who "tries" to be supportive, but really is negative, critical, or judgmental instead. Then begin to use your walking meditation to protect you from any negative energy that these well-meaning but misguided people send your way.

To help you keep on track throughout your day, print out this short list, and check often to see if you're nurturing your will power with your attitudes and actions.

Create a definite purpose, and build it into a compelling desire.

Create a specific plan, and check each day to make sure you're following it.

Don't accept any negative or discouraging suggestions, from others or from yourself.

Join with others to nurture and encourage each other.

From sugar to fruit

Now it's time to start re-training your mind to think "fruit" and "salad" instead of candy, cake, donuts, and soft drinks. Any time you feel the need for something sweet you will probably get a thought that says "candy"(or something equally dangerous.)

Gently move that thought out of your mind, and get yourself an apple, an orange, some strawberries, or a large, tasty salad. Make sure that you plan ahead so that you always have at least four pieces of fruit to eat throughout the day.

This is what your body really needs, and is the underlying cause of the craving for something sweet. Feed your body what it is really telling you it needs, so that you can begin to repair the damage caused by all those years of sugar and fat consumption.

Remember that old saying —"All things in moderation"? I remember years ago my mother's best friend, Edna, was told by her doctor that she could eat all the fruit she wanted. Edna weighed over 300 pounds, and her doctor was seriously worried about her heart.

The next time Edna went to the doctor, she weighed even more than she had before. Why? She had taken the doctor literally — and was now eating a box of oranges every day!

That's why it's important to remember that fruits aren't the only thing our sweet tooth is trying to lead us to. The most healthful foods, in addition to fruit, are the sweet-tasting leaves — like lettuce, kale, chard and spinach, as well as vegetables like broccoli, peas and beans. Sweet potatoes, squash, and zucchini are also sweet. But only taste sweet after you've kicked the sugar habit.

You truly can eat as much as you want of the green salads and steamed vegetables that taste so good. Even Edna would have lost weight if her doctor had told her to eat as much salad as she wanted (without high-fat dressings, of course.) Your taste buds will quickly adapt to the lower sugar levels, and you'll find yourself craving fruits, salads and beans.

It may seem impossible now, while you're still hooked on sugar, but remember — your body never really wanted that sugar. It wanted the nutrients that come packaged in sweet fruits and vegetables. Once your body recognizes that it is finally getting all the nutrients it was starving for, your cravings will change.

We naturally associate obesity with the consumption of large quantities of food — so it's sometimes hard to realize that this is a disease of malnutrition.

If you feel a desire for fruit, but misread that appetite and feed it a candy bar instead, your body will be getting empty calories that do absolutely nothing for your health. While those calories can be burned, like firewood in a stove, they can't build the body's cells, keep the immune system working, or add to your general well-being.

So, naturally, your survival system will tell you to eat more food, and give you the hint that it should be sweet. Your body is starving for the nutrients packed in plants, but our modern technology has found a way to suck the pure calories out of sugar beets, leaving all the nutrients behind.

Sugar builds corporation profits — it doesn't build bodies.

Once your body is no longer starving for nutrients, your cravings will naturally subside. That doesn't mean that your appetite for sweetness will go away — that will never happen. It's part of your survival system, so you wouldn't want it to.

To learn more about your body's nutritional needs, be sure to read the book *Eat to Live: The Revolutionary Formula for Fast and Sustained Weight Loss*. It will help you learn to read your body correctly, and replace the bad food with miracle food. You don't have to eat less — you just have to eat right.

What happens when you go "cold turkey" and give up sugar and other refined carbohydrates?

You will go through a short period of withdrawal, much like an alcoholic when he gives up his booze. However, your withdrawal symptoms will not be life-threatening — it's just a period of discomfort while your body busies itself with detoxifying your cells.

Oddly enough, few people have any withdrawal symptoms when they drastically reduce the fat in their diets. Sugar appears to be physically addictive, while fat and salt become habits because we get used to the taste. When we re-train our taste buds to enjoy natural, healthy food, our bodies celebrate. You may miss the taste of your favorite high-fat, high-salt food, but your body won't miss them at all.

To keep from feeling picked on while you change over to your new diet, remember that the slight discomfort you feel is not your body trying to get you to go back to sugar and fat. It is your body getting rid of the years of accumulated toxins. It is unfortunate, but you will need to go through this period of feeling worse, before you can feel better. It doesn't take long — a week or two at the most.

Keep up your walking meditation, and eat a varied diet filled with fruits and vegetables — Dr. Fuhrman wants you to include a huge salad with every lunch and dinner, so that you get all the phytochemicals you need to rebuild your body's immune system. It also gives you the fiber that helps wash the excess fat out of your body.

We hear so much about calories that we assume that every extra fat molecule in our body has to be burned with exercise and sweat in order to lose weight. Actually, your body dislikes all those fat cells as much as you do. When you begin to give your body lots of fruits, salads, vegetables and beans, it will have the energy it needs to begin scouring out all that excess, toxic fat. Your extra weight will fall away, even if you aren't able to exercise the way you feel you should.

Are you home free? Well, you've made a wonderful start. Keep up your walking meditation, continue to read about nutrition and health, and stay focused on your new dietary goals. As soon as you give up sugar and fat, your weight will begin to drop dramatically, and that will be a wonderful incentive to keep on your program. But the mind works in mysterious ways, and there still may be roadblocks along the way.

There is one thing, chronic stress, that can make walking meditation extremely difficult to practice and master — and it also makes it very hard to rise above our habitual responses to food or anything else. In the next chapter we'll see why stress makes dieting so difficult, and learn how you can use walking meditation to reduce the stress in your life.

Action Step #5

Is it an obstacle, or an excuse? How do you tell the difference?

We all know how other people can sometimes complain or gripe about the same darn thing over and over again — but never do anything to fix the problem.

But it's really hard to see it when we do it ourselves. It's just human nature.

In order to really look at your thoughts, so you can clearly see if you are voicing true obstacles, or just nurturing excuses that prevent action, print out the following page and answer the questions honestly.

Then sleep on it, as you've done with the previous Action Steps. For this particular step you may actually need the help of a friend or loved one who is brave enough to be honest with you.

Here's the purpose of this exercise. You'll write down every statement you can remember making in the last week or month for not doing something. Did someone make a suggestion that you rejected? Did you find yourself ignoring some of the steps in this book? Did you complain about something at work or at home?

Write it down, whether it has anything to do with your diet or not. It really doesn't matter, since this is an exercise in really seeing your thoughts, and finding out whether or not they lead you closer to your goals. And you have lots of goals in your life, don't you?

Once you've written your list of excuses (or reasons, if that's the case) ask yourself how many times you've repeated that particular statement, or called on that particular excuse for not making a change.

If the number is greater than two, and yet you have yet to sit down and create a plan for overcoming this problem, it is probable that you are leaning on an excuse, rather than discussing an obstacle. Obstacles can be walked around, or over. They can be moved out of the way. If the obstacle is big enough, you can get your friends together to help.

But excuses just sit there, keeping you paralyzed with inaction. So be honest with yourself. You want to change —don't let your own thoughts stop you from getting what you want.

Chronic stress

I have a friend who has told me at least once a week for the last four years that she is "almost ready" to start a weight-loss program. Her doctor has warned her that her blood pressure and cholesterol levels are dangerously high. And she tells me the things she has done in the past to lose weight and regain her energy and vitality.

She obviously has all the knowledge she needs in order to start on a good weight loss program. But nothing happens.

I'm sure you also know people who want to be thin and healthy, and who have a strong wish to have the vitality and health that they remember from the past. It's possible that they aren't changing, even though they want to, because they're living with chronic, self-induced stress.

This may also be true for you. If your mind is full of negative memories and angry or anxious thoughts, many of your eating choices will be made by your instinctual mind, because it believes you're in constant, unfocused danger. This makes it difficult to replace your habitual diet with the healthy fruits and vegetables your body needs.

Why does stress make it more difficult to lose weight?

Your instinctual mind naturally believes it should be in charge when you are thinking about what to eat, because food is necessary for your survival.

The instinctual mind will also take over when it believes itself to be in danger.

Because you have spent years equating the instinctual need for sweetness with sugar and other fattening foods, stress is a double threat to our success with a weight loss program. This is especially true during the first few months when you are working hard to overcome your addiction to sugar.

When it perceives a threat, the brain causes the adrenal glands to release chemicals into the body that are very similar in structure and effect to amphetamine and opium. These chemicals prepare the body for that famous "fight or flight" behavior that is a natural response to danger.

While those chemicals are coursing through your body, you will make instinctive (and therefore instantaneous) decisions. If there is a real emergency, this is good – it could even save your life.

If you live under chronic stress, you have these same chemicals in your body all of the time. You may even have become addicted to them. As long as the stress chemicals are kept at abnormally high levels, the instinctual mind will fight for control, because it believes your survival is at stake.

This is the reason why it is so difficult to change our lives while we live in chronic stress. People living with chronic stress spend a lot of brain power making up and maintaining excuses for decisions they have not consciously made, leaving little energy left for change.

If you are one of the many people who are living in a chronically stressful environment, you will need to learn to recognize which stress is coming from the outside, and which stress is actually coming from the way you think – and is therefore subject to change.

But what if the stress comes from real danger?

Many nutritional experts and diet book authors, including Dr. Henry Mallek (who wrote *The New Longevity Diet*), believe that if our environment is truly chaotic (or even dangerous), we need to get our lives in order and remove the external sources of stress before we can even begin to think about becoming successful with a weight loss or nutritional program.

I have to disagree with them.

There is one aspect of your life that cannot be controlled by anyone but you - what you choose to put in your mouth. Because what you eat may be just about the only thing you can do that does not appear to be controlled by outside circumstances or other people, I believe that your commitment to lose weight is even more important. Not just to give you a better body, but to give you some of the skills that you need in order to take more control of your life.

Think of each eating choice as an opportunity to create a moment of strength in a day filled with unhappiness or fear. Allow yourself the right to "wake up." even for just one moment, and put your conscious mind in charge of this one small piece of your life.

By nurturing those few moments, and honoring them, the conscious mind begins to grow stronger. You become more and more "yourself" - and at the same time, you get slimmer and healthier. It may even give you the strength to make that phone call and get the help you know you need.

Clearly, this book is not intended to "fix" your situation, to save the world, to change human nature. It's just about learning how to keep your commitment to lose weight and become healthier. So, if you need help from a therapist, a doctor, or even a women's shelter or crisis line, please make that phone call, and get what you need.

What if you're depressed or compulsive?

Sometimes the thoughts in our minds seem almost uncontrollable. If you feel this is true, you may have been stressed out for so long that you now have a chemical imbalance that affects your mind's ability to control your thoughts.

Depression is usually thought of as a way that people feel, but it does affect your thoughts and your decisions, too. It is considered a form of mental illness, because it is associated with processes and chemicals in the brain. The same thing is true of obsessive/compulsive disorder.

Many people avoid seeking treatment for depression and obsessive/compulsive disorders because they fear that they will need to be medicated forever. While this is something that you would need to discuss with your doctor, it is also possible that a short time on prescription medication could give you the "window of opportunity" that you need in order to calm down and begin a program that gives you more control over your thoughts.

Prolonged, repetitive negative thoughts can cause depression, in much the same way that amphetamine use can if it is extended over a long period of time. Because of the affect that depression has on your thought processes, it makes it difficult to follow any self-help program. So if this is a problem for you, talk to your doctor — she really may be able to help.

Then begin to practice the walking meditation and other mental exercises in this book so that you can learn to reduce your stress naturally, and begin to take back control of your thoughts, your eating program, and your life. A healthy eating program filled with fruits and vegetables can also help you feel stronger and more energetic, which helps you feel less depressed.

If you're not quite ready for medical intervention, but you are still too stressed or depressed to practice walking meditation, you might want to consider listening to the Sedona Tapes. They have been shown in a number of studies to reduce stress and help to control depression. While they are a bit expensive, they may be what you need in order to get back in control. Your doctor can help you decide if this option is right for you.

Whatever you choose to do, remember — your instinctive mind will have the upper hand if you are living in chronic stress, but there are ways to regain control of the thoughts that cause the chronic stress in many lives. For many people, the mental exercises in the next chapter, when practiced along with walking meditation, can make a huge difference.

Taking control

Do you have a friend who fully intends to lose weight but just hasn't yet gotten around to it? It's possible that chronic stress allows her unconscious mind to make many of her eating decisions for her.

She's literally pulled in two different directions. She wants to eat better, but she doesn't. She wants to lose 20 or 30 pounds, but she doesn't. She wants to walk every day to give herself the exercise she knows she needs, but she doesn't do it.

A few years ago I was in exactly the same place. I had experienced the loss of a marriage and the death of my mother, and for a full year my mind was filled with negative memories. I spent more time living inside those negative memories than I did in the real world. Many spiritual masters would say I was "asleep." And it tended to be a nightmare.

There were so many things I wanted to accomplish, but I spent almost all of my mental energy on the negative thoughts inside my mind. They were like angry, frustrating movies replayed over and over and over again.

I hated those movies. But I didn't know how to turn them off. In fact, it didn't even occur to me that it was possible.

Then I read *Psycho-Pictography: The New Way to Use the Miracle Power of Your Mind,* by Vernon Howard (one of my all-time favorite books, and it's recently become unavailable!) which told me that I could actually choose what I thought about. Strange as it may sound, it had never occurred to me. That discovery was the basis for the system I outline in this book, which has literally changed my life.

Now that you, too, are practicing walking meditation, perhaps you've also noticed yourself replaying endless repetitions of the same negative events over and over. If this is happening, you are probably living in constant, chronic stress that is actually created by this repetitive "tape" inside your mind.

This has a huge effect on your ability to reach your weight loss goals. If you are watching negative movies in your head, the stress it creates will allow your unconscious mind to be in charge of your decisions far more often than you had ever realized. This makes it much easier to believe those false thoughts that lead you back into addictions to unhealthy food.

The repetitive negative thoughts that occupy many people's minds can sap a huge percentage of their daily allotment of energy, leaving them drained and unable to make the conscious decisions that would bring about useful change. For many of us, the first decisions that get "taken over" by the unconscious mind are the ones involving food!

Try this experiment:

Go for a walk and intentionally think about an event in your life that brings you anxiety or unhappiness. Remember it in full detail, the way you do when you daydream. At a certain prearranged point in your walk, begin to think about a very happy memory — some event that gave you great joy and comfort. Or even think of an exciting event that you have planned for the future.

Now, notice that you are walking faster!

When I walk down a city street thinking about a very happy or interesting thought, I find that I actually am walking faster than people who are much younger than I am. When we let go of our negative memories, we have much more energy for the things in life that we really want. The reduction in stress also takes away our survival system's need to stay in control and make decisions for us.

Why do negative thoughts add to your stress?

Every emotionally charged picture that we put into our minds is believed to be true, at that moment, by our instinctive self, which governs our emotions.

While the instinctual mind cannot understand words, abstract thoughts, or most ideas, it does respond to emotionally charged internal pictures — but not in the way we might expect. "Imaginary" is an abstract thought, after all, and the instinctual mind cannot know if the picture it sees is part of a memory, or a Hollywood movie, or a real event happening now.

So it believes every emotionally charged picture it sees is happening now, and reacts accordingly. That reaction is the immediate release of the chemicals that put us into fight or flight status — even when there's nothing to run from, or to fight with. And this leads to chronic stress.

Why is it so hard to realize that we're causing ourselves stress with our thoughts?

Let's look at how our "old brain" reacts to movies at a theater, and how it is different from our reaction to the pictures we see inside our minds in the form of thoughts and daydreams. The emotions that are created, and the chemical response, are actually the same — but our awareness of the process is different.

Every good novel and every exciting movie capitalizes on our bodies' ability to feel the emotions that are appropriate for the story we hear or see. Intense emotional responses feel good (even when the emotion is anger), which is why we pay so much money to watch and read stories that help us feel strong emotions. Steven Spielberg has made millions because of this instinctual response.

During a movie our instinctive mind believes the pictures on the screen, and reacts emotionally to them, even though our conscious mind knows we are just watching a movie. When we walk out of the theater, the pictures have disappeared, so the instinctive mind no longer has any "danger" or "loss" to respond to, and the body's chemical balance goes back to normal.

We get an emotional rush that feels good in the movie theater because of the chemicals that are created by the body in response to danger, fear or loss. As we learned before, those chemicals are very similar in structure and effect to amphetamines and opium. When they come in short doses, during a real emergency or during a movie, they have no harmful effects. It is the chronic "use" of these chemicals that is destructive to our bodies and minds.

When we tell ourselves an emotionally charged story (in the form of a thought or memory or daydream), our instinctive mind "believes" the pictures it sees in our imagination as though the event we are thinking about were actually happening now — and we re-experience the feelings of anger or disappointment that we felt when the event was actually taking place.

Then, our conscious mind notices that we are now experiencing anger or some other strong emotion, and we believe that this feeling is being caused by the original event, when it is actually being caused by replaying a picture of the event inside our mind.

There have been times in my life when I have been absolutely convinced that some past insult or loss was terribly important to me, simply because I was able to continue feeling the anger or loss for such a long time after the event was over. I was actually manufacturing those negative emotions by replaying the memory of past events over and over again. And I was certainly not aware of the fact that I could turn off the internal movie.

I was hooked on the chemicals that I was creating in response to my manufactured stress (and they are addictive)! so my unconscious mind kept repeating the negative memories over and over again, in order to get the rush. I didn't want to keep repeating those scenes any longer, but until I learned to practice walking meditation I didn't know that I had the power to stop.

And, as we learned earlier, the chronic stress that comes from repeated negative imagery will keep the survival system in power. That means that the instinctual mind will be making choices for you when you don't realize it — making it extremely difficult to succeed in taking control and losing weight.

One way to know if you are unconsciously using negative thoughts in order to create this "rush" of emotions is to watch your thoughts — walking meditation.

Here's another exercise that also works, because it helps you notice your thoughts at times when you aren't specifically working on controlling them. This gives you a great indication of what it is that you think about habitually — and to see if those thoughts are adding to your stress.

The next time you are out driving, decide in advance that each time you come to a stop light, or pass a red car, you'll notice what you are thinking about. It's a way of "checking in" and seeing what's going on inside your mind.

When you notice that you are thinking or daydreaming about something that made you angry or sad in the past, be sure to also notice that you are now feeling angry or sad — in response to the pictures you have put in your mind. And notice that those negative emotions, which sap so much of your energy, will go away as soon as you focus on something else.

Many people are amazed to find that they are "addicted" to negative thoughts. If you find yourself thinking about something that causes you to feel some powerful emotion now, even though the event happened in the past, you may be "deliberately" flooding your body with the natural equivalents of speed and opium. Strange as it sounds, your unconscious mind is making you feel bad on purpose!

No matter how long you may have been stressing yourself out with negative thoughts, you can change your mental habits and reduce the stress.

You will use the skills you've gained during walking meditation. As you find yourself thinking about an argument last week, simply say to yourself that you've already experienced that particular scene, thank you very much, and would prefer to think about something different.

Then choose to replace this thought with a memory of success or an exciting plan for the future. You will be able to feel your blood pressure going down within seconds. This is a very powerful skill that you are learning.

When I first learned this technique I coined a phrase that helped me to stay on track. That phrase is "A rabbit doesn't run from yesterday's fox."

What this means is that if you are feeling an emotion now because of something that happened yesterday or last year; if you're nursing a grudge that should have been abandoned a long time ago; or if you're obsessively remembering a loss that you cannot replace; you are using precious resources that could be better spent on the challenges you face today.

When you find yourself running from yesterday's fox, use your walking meditation skills, and choose to think about something else.

It is important to remember that it is emotionally charged stories that the instinctive mind responds to. And the emotions of joy, love, excitement and anticipation can replace the negative emotions of fear and loss — if we choose to remember and dream about events that include those positive feelings.

What does all this have to do with "thinking thin"?

Imagine it — you will soon be able to turn aside an emotionally charged daydream that has been following you around for weeks. You won't do this by arguing with your thoughts, or even listening to your excuses. You'll simply choose to think something else.

Now imagine yourself in a cafeteria line, looking at the overhead menu board. You came with the intention of getting a salad, but the hamburger is calling you. You start wanting that hamburger, and it seems like nothing else will do.

Notice the thought, set it aside, and replace it with the words "I'll have the salad, please." No argument, no stress, no inner turmoil — and no hamburger on your plate. You'll have everything you need to be successful with your diet.

It will be so easy, it will feel like magic.

Action Step #6

One of the most difficult things to do is give up negative, repetitive thoughts. We almost seem to need them, as though they were old friends. But as you've seen, negative thoughts actually change the chemistry of your brain, and make change almost impossible.

For that reason, it helps to start writing down each memory or repetitive thought as it comes to you. Many times, these negative thoughts are the same as the excuses that you wrote down in Action Step #5 — but there are other thoughts that you also need to be aware of.

Is there a particular event in the recent or ancient past that you dwell on? Is there a particular family member or old friend who did or said something that you still haven't forgiven her for? Do you still feel jittery or mildly upset every time you think of what someone said, or what someone did, yesterday or last week or last year?

When you feel your blood pressure going up, or notice a mild or deep anxiety about something, remember the rule:

"A rabbit doesn't run from yesterday's fox."

If it isn't happening now, right this minute, your brain is creating a damaging emotion by visualizing an image that your subconscious brain believes to be real. But you know it isn't real.

Even if you are intensely attached to a grudge, memory or discontent, write it down so that you can make a conscious choice — do you allow it to keep you mired in doubt, anxiety and defeat, or do you let it go so you can make the changes you want so much?

Go ahead and start writing.

Learn to love yourself

I almost put this chapter first, because the meditation I describe here is so powerful. It is amazing how a simple guided daydream can help us do what so many experts tell us we need to do — but without telling us how!

You've read the books — about relationships, parenting, career success, and weight loss — that tell you that you need to love yourself before doing anything else. They say that it will set the stage for a frame of mind that can help you feel confident and secure, because you know you will get support and hugs from the one person who knows you best — you!

When you practice this simple mental exercise you will not only feel what it is like to love yourself, you will also find yourself more relaxed and more confident.

And that means you can more easily stay in control of your eating choices. You don't need to practice this meditation, but it feels so good, you'll be glad you did.

It's not about self-esteem.

Can we learn to love ourselves by telling ourselves how nice or good or beautiful we are, as though we were trying to help a child gain self-esteem?

You can try, but it probably won't change the way you feel about yourself. When you tell yourself you're a nice

70

person, or smart, or beautiful, or successful, you are actually offering yourself a judgment. True, it is a positive judgment, which is better than a negative one. But love and approval are not the same thing.

All of us crave the kind of love that is really only possible when we're infants. We want to be accepted and cared for without judgment of any kind. We want to be enveloped with the feeling of safety that comes from a parent who is completely devoted to our needs and who truly enjoys our company.

In time, of course, we have to grow up. Our behavior and our accomplishments do matter to the people around us. And we become the parent who gives that unconditional love (for a while) to our own children. But we still crave the wonderful, warm, feel-good experience that few of us can ever re-create in real life in the completeness that we desire.

Some people replace that feeling with food. "Emotional eating" may be less common than we think. Many of us eat from addiction, and call it emotion. Nonetheless, "comfort food" has a huge appeal, and this exercise (along with a healthy diet full of the life-giving fruits and vegetables our body needs), can help cut down on the need to eat to feel loved.

Before we begin this powerful exercise, let's see how it feels to not love ourselves. We'll do it through mental imagery. Think of it as a guided daydream — and have fun with it!

Relax for a moment, and imagine the following scene. You're walking in your favorite place, perhaps along a deserted beach or high on a mesa in the Arizona desert. Your only companion is a wolf (or cougar, or eagle). It doesn't really matter what kind of animal it is — you have your own favorite wild beast, so choose whichever one you like.

This companion is both your friend and your protector. You are comfortable in each other's presence, and rely on each other for support and companionship. You love watching her move her beautiful body so effortlessly. Watch her ears move as she hears birds or mice, see the different ways she expresses her interest in things, and her emotions. Imagine that this is something that you do every day, and that nothing could be more natural.

Enjoy your walk for as long as you like, and then stop for a moment and sit on a rock or log. Just enjoy the fresh air and the solitude in this wonderful place. Let your companion come sit beside you, perhaps resting her chin on your knee. Stroke her soft, silky fur, and scratch her just behind the ears. You know the special spot that makes her happy.

Know that you and your companion are completely at peace, and love each other.

Now suddenly you jump up, wave your arms around wildly and start yelling angrily — it doesn't matter why. Your companion is frightened, and runs. She doesn't run far, because she needs you, but the trust is broken. She cowers away from you, in fear and anger. Peace has disappeared.

It feels lonely, doesn't it — as though you have lost a connection that had become important to you?

The first time a friend used this guided daydream, it made her cry because the loss felt so real.

If you have an internal judge (and who doesn't)? you may feel this type of internal division, which prevents you from loving yourself without judgment. But we can now change that, simply by taking the term "love yourself" literally.

Think back to a time when you felt really loved. You may remember a hug or a warm look or a gift that showed you that someone truly enjoyed being with you. You felt warm and cared for. And someone else was there with you, even if it was someone of a different species, such as a dog or cat.

Love is a felt connection between two beings.

And there is only one of you. So how can you love yourself? (Actually, the same way you get angry at yourself, but you already know how to do that, don't you?) To feel what it is like to be loved unconditionally, you need to bring an image into your mind of a situation in which you are loved. Since love requires two parties, you need to imagine the "other" you that loves you.

You can do this by imagining yourself as that guardian animal that was in the first meditation, or you can replace her with a picture of yourself at a time in your life when you really needed a hug from someone who understood and valued you.

This "division" of yourself for the purposes of this exercise may seem silly while you read about it, but do try this meditation — it will create the feeling of being loved (by yourself) — and you can use the memory of that feeling any time you need an emotional hug. Remember — any emotionally charged story is believed by your unconscious, so you will literally feel loved. What a nice way to spend a few moments.

Because this meditation is so powerful, you should prepare your environment so that you can really relax and enjoy it. You may even choose to tape this story, and take it with you so that you aren't distracted by having to read it. You'll need to be in a place with no distractions or other people — so find a nice comfy place where you can be alone.

Now that you are very comfortable and calm, close your eyes and bring into your mind a picture of yourself in that special place that you imagined at the beginning of this chapter. Your companion animal is still there, still cowering and lacking trust. (Remember, you can replace her with an image of yourself, if you like.)

Take a second to bring back the image of that place, with the feeling of the air, the sound in the trees. And remember the feeling of loss you felt when your companion ran away from you in fear.

Now you have a chance to take the time to do whatever is needed to bring back the trust that was lost between you. Lower yourself to your heels, hold out your hand, and speak slowly and softly. Remember, give it time, and go slowly.

Put yourself completely into this scene, by imagining the feel of the air against your skin, the bark or sand beneath your feet, and the sound of birds or waves. Make it as real as you can — really feel the story.

Before long, your companion will slowly come towards you, tentatively at first. Be sure to stay calm so that she can relax her guard.

Is she back by your side? Good. Take a minute to feel calm, and watch her slowly become more trustful. As you stay calm, she'll forget her previous scare, and want to play again.

Now, go for a walk, or play a game, or just enjoy being with her. You know that your companion is happy to be back with you. How does she show her happiness? Does she lean against you, or run about in excitement? Does she bring you sticks and shells that she finds on the ground? Keep seeing this picture until you really feel loved at this moment. Enjoy the feeling.

Go fully into the meditation, and stay there for as long as it is comfortable. When you feel a need to come back out of your daydream, there is one thing you should do first.

Call your companion toward you, stroke her head and become totally focused on the love and trust that you share with her. Then imagine that she slowly turns into a ball of light, which you can hold in your cupped hands. Bring this beautiful glowing energy toward you, and let it enter your chest — then let it diffuse throughout your body, your arms and legs and toes. Feel the warmth of this energy for a few moments before you slowly come back to the here-and-now.

Wow — do you now feel calmer, more in control, more confident? You have just learned how to love yourself.

If you have just read the story, and haven't really taken the time to imagine it fully, close your eyes and do it now. Try it. It feels good.

You can actually use this daydream to resolve some of the pain you are still holding on to from the past. Imagine yourself, as a child or younger adult, at a time when you really felt the need for someone's love and support. Now enter the scene as yourself — at your present age, and give your imaginary younger self a hug. Stay with her and let her explain why she was frightened, or lonely, or sad. It can be a wonderful tool for self-healing.

If you are in a stressful situation at work or home, and don't have much time, you can still use your imagination to reduce your stress level. Just imagine your imaginary "other self" giving you a hug. It only takes a few seconds and your blood pressure will go down. Looking at a piece of chocolate cake and need some extra strength to walk away from it? Imagine your "self" taking your hand and leading you to that juicy orange, instead. Sure, it seems a bit weird — but it helps, so why not?

If you replace negative memories with this daydream of you loving yourself, you will be replacing fear, anger, grief and loss with love, support, and companionship. The negative memories will come less often, they'll have less power, and you'll experience far less chronic stress.

You've learned some incredibly powerful skills in the last few chapters. You're now able to notice thoughts as they come into your mind, and gently replace them with thoughts of your own choosing. You now have control, even over powerful thoughts about food. You know what it's like to be "awake" and you feel more confident and more in control.

Since you are just starting out on this new journey, the next chapter shows you some easy, fun "tricks" to use while you're building your new skills. And we'll also look at exactly how to use your skills when faced with that tempting donut.

Action Step #7

When I was writing this book, I noticed something that happens a lot — when we talk about dieting, or changing the way we eat, many of us begin to think and speak like children. Not too long ago, I was as guilty of this as anyone.

What do I mean by "thinking like children?"

When you eat a candy bar or anything else that you've placed on your list of things to avoid eating, why do you call it "cheating"? Who is it that you're hiding it from? If you don't get caught by that someone, what, exactly, are you getting away with?

Cheating is something that children aren't supposed to do when they take a test. And when they get caught, we hope that we can keep them from doing it again by making them feel guilty.

Trust me — guilt has no place in the Weight Loss: How to Keep Your Commitment program.

Many people also feel "picked on" when they can't eat the way they were used to, even though they've chosen to eat a new and healthy diet because it's good for them.

Anytime you feel "picked on," or find yourself plotting about how to get away with cheating on your diet — you know that your addiction is at work, creating the kind of false thoughts that Alcoholics Anonymous calls "stinking thinking."

It's time to move away from those self-defeating thoughts, and make conscious, healthy decisions.

I'm absolutely convinced that the concept of "cheating" (and the acceptance of the idea that diets are a form of denial that naturally leaves us feeling picked on) is far more destructive than eating one candy bar or one hamburger possibly could be.

That way of thinking sets you up for failure.

Think about a person who you admire, someone who has achieved the things you only dream about. Does that person spend any precious time plotting and scheming about how she'll "get away" with doing something that moves her away from her own goals?

Does he pout when someone mentions a promise that he made to himself?

Have you read any book about success in business or any other aspect of life that listed "guilt" as one of the cornerstones for success?

When diet books say that a good attitude is the most important thing you need to be successful on a diet, they're absolutely right. A good attitude is the basis of any success, whether the goal is related to health, or family, or relationships, or career.

The best books to read for inspiration when you're beginning a new diet are actually not diet books — they're great works by the masters of success. Read your favorite spiritual leader, or read the words of one of today's top marketing or business speakers. These are the folks who really understand what makes for a "good attitude"!

One person whose words you should read is Napoleon Hill. Mr. Hill wrote the classic book *Think & Grow Rich*. I want you to read a short excerpt from this small book, which has changed the lives of thousands of people who were willing (and able) to learn from it:

> When Henley wrote the prophetic lines, "I am the master of my fate, I am the captain of my soul," he should have informed us that we are the masters of our fate, the captains of our souls, because we have the power to control our thoughts.
>
> He should have told us that our brains become magnetized with the dominating thoughts which we hold in our minds, and, by means with which no man is familiar, these "magnets" attract to us the forces, the people, the circumstances of life which harmonize with the nature of our dominating thoughts.

If your thoughts are dominated by ideas about "cheating" and being "picked on," imagine what that is doing to your commitment to your own happiness and health! If you're spending any mental energy on thinking up ways to get away with doing something that is not in your own best interest, it's time to do some very serious soul searching.

One of the most important habits to learn is to celebrate every success, and analyze every defeat — and then move on. But "cheating" isn't really a "defeat" if it's caused by intentional self-sabotage. We can't learn anything from the fact that we managed to shoot ourselves in the foot, just as we intended to.

But you can learn from true slips in your diet. In fact, after a while you actually welcome these slips because

78

they allow you to know yourself better, and really get in tune with what your body needs.

Start noticing any time you begin to think about acting outside your plan, and ask yourself if that really helps you achieve your dream of losing weight and getting healthy? If the answer is no, you've just found a perfect opportunity to use the skills you gained, walking meditation. You know the drill — choose to think about something else.

Now what?

Have you always associated weight-loss with a struggle, a fight, a constant battle? Now you know it doesn't have to be that way.

How do you really use walking meditation in order to help you lose weight? Remember, a successful weight-loss program requires the right choices. Whether or not those choices are made by the instinctual or your conscious mind is totally dependent upon your being "awake" when that choice is being made.

How long does it take to decide between a donut and a salad? Just a few seconds, right? Those are the few seconds when you need to be awake, and take control.

Do you fight with yourself, feeling as though a battle is being waged inside your head? The instinctual mind has made its choice (donut) and your conscious mind is building the immediate excuse for that decision (you didn't have time for breakfast, just one won't hurt, everyone else is having one, etc...), even though you are committed to staying on your diet.

Your awareness switches quickly from two opposing statements — "it's OK to eat the donut," and "it's absolutely imperative that you not eat the donut. " You are of two minds.

If you continue the argument, you will lose (your commitment will lose) because your instinctual mind isn't participating in the conversation. Its decision has already been made. You are arguing with the excuse for that decision, which has no basis in fact at all. It is an automatic response to an instinctual decision, and has no validity whatsoever.

While you are spending all that energy debating with yourself, your hand will simply reach out and select your favorite pastry. And then you'll beat yourself up for giving in to your drive for sugar and fat. After you've practiced walking meditation long enough, you will be able to simply move the "wrong" thought out of your mind, and regain all that energy that you would have spent on arguing with it.

I know that you already have all the decision-making skills that you need to make the right eating choices, as long as you're fully conscious. How can I be so sure? Because you make hundreds of decisions every single day, and the vast majority of those decisions are made with no internal argument or struggle at all

How to back up from an emotional situation.

In the beginning of your "think thin" program, your instinctual self is still trying very hard to stay in control of this part of your life — so your emotions are engaged during a struggle over food. In an emotional situation, it is difficult to back up and make a simple, conscious choice that goes against your natural drive to eat badly. For this reason, I personally found it helpful to also use several "tricks" while I was still fairly new to the practice of walking meditation.

I found the first trick I used in books about Neuro-linguistic Programming. This trick can actually be fun, and helps you to "back away" from your emotional involvement so that you can make a conscious decision about food — or anything else that has a high emotional charge.

Don't wait until you are actually faced with one of those situations where you know you are likely to go off your diet. Practice the method in advance, in a nice quiet place where you can really pay attention to how you feel.

First, imagine one of those tempting situations as clearly as you can. You've been in many of them in the past, so remembering one won't be hard. One situation that most of us can easily imagine is the family gathering, where everyone competes to bring the tastiest, and most fattening, food to lovingly share. All your favorite food from your childhood is laid out on the buffet table, whispering "just this once won't hurt..."

Bring into your mind an image that is as clear as you can muster — including the tempting food, the social situation, the room you're in, the smell of the food — everything. You will feel emotionally torn between accepting the food that you know isn't good for you, and wanting to walk away from it.

To get away from that emotionality, I now want you to imagine that you are watching exactly the same scene, but as it appears on a movie screen. You are in one of the seats in the theater, watching yourself struggle with the decision of what to eat. Pay very close attention to how it feels to watch yourself in that situation. If you feel any emotional connection at all, you are still too close to it and need to back up even further.

If that is the case, move into the projection booth, and watch yourself sitting in the theater, watching the movie. By now the whole scene should have lost all emotionalism and has probably moved into the absurd. That's exactly where you want it!

Now, as you stand in the projection booth, how would you have the "you" on the screen act? It's your movie, so go ahead and write the script any way you want!

Is your hostess handing you a plate filled with two kinds of cake and a piece of Aunt Betty's famous fudge brownie? Imagine yourself taking the plate, saying thank you, and then setting the plate down somewhere and "forgetting" about it. Are you at a company potluck? Imagine yourself filling your plate with the lettuce, tomatoes and other veggie trim that is intended to top those fat-filled grilled hamburgers.

Go ahead and fill in all the details, watching yourself make that appropriate, conscious decision. The more you practice this mental imagery, the more strength you will have when you are actually faced with the situation in real life.

This is a variation of the technique that world-class athletes use when they practice their moves in their minds. It has been proven that if you practice free-throws in your head you will make more accurate shots the next time you're on the court. Your imagination is a very powerful tool, if you use it for positive change.

Creating an alter-ego to blame for your "stinking thinking."

I'll let you in on another trick I used whenever I noticed a thought had come into my mind that was telling me that I couldn't do what I wanted. This one is very good to use when your own mind is trying to talk you out of something, such as going for a walk or spending some time in the gym. (I still have to drag my little demon out on cold mornings when I'd rather sleep in than work out.)

Once I had practiced noticing my thoughts, I was amazed at how sneaky my instinctual mind could be. This reminded me of one of my favorite cartoon characters — the Coyote in the Roadrunner cartoons. And this gave me an idea...

I knew my instinctive mind really believed it was making the best choice for me, but was simply mistaken. Since the negative excuse was actually manufactured by my conscious mind to explain that mistaken choice, it would do no good to argue with the excuse. But I needed a way to reduce its power in the present moment — when it was telling me that I couldn't have what I wanted.

So I built an image in my mind to represent the negative thoughts, as though they were coming from someone else. (This is very similar to the approached used by an addictions self-help organization called SMART Recovery®.)

I created a little elf-like creature that had the cartoon Coyote's miraculous ability to withstand incredible punishment without any permanent harm. Then, when a thought popped into my mind that said I couldn't have what I wanted, or do what I had chosen to do, I imagined myself grabbing that little guy and pounding away on him.

I made my little scene totally excessive, like the Roadrunner cartoon, so it was funny. And because I knew he would pop up again the next time he wanted to stop me from doing something, there was no way anything I imagined could do my little demon any lasting harm. I didn't have to feel guilty.

Try this the next time you find yourself wanting to do something that is counter to your weight-loss goals. Perhaps your coworkers have brought in donuts as a reward for some major project your group has completed at work, and they put the box of donuts on a table right next to your desk. (I didn't have to make up this scene – it happens all the time where I work.)

If you hear yourself thinking that "just one won't hurt," grab your imaginary little guy and beat the crap out of him. Make up whatever scene you will think is funny. The only thing your coworkers will notice is that you are smiling when you say "no thanks! "

Make sure to notice when you are most vulnerable.

As you become more and more aware of the times when you find yourself making excuses and filling your mind with "stinking thinking, " as the folks at Alcoholics Anonymous call it, you can begin to see patterns in your day when stress is unusually high or when you are tired.

These are the times when you are most vulnerable to making bad eating choices based on instinct. When you have become conscious of these patterns, you can then make changes in your day to reduce that stress and give your commitment to weight loss and good health a better chance for success.

How can you tell if your conscious mind is in control?

How do you know if you've made a conscious choice from the restaurant menu, or if you're just making an excuse for an instinctive choice?

A conscious choice and an instinctual choice will look very much the same when you look at them in your mind. The only way you can really know if you are making the right choice is to compare the expected results of that choice against the results you want.

Excuses almost never take your long-term goals into account.

Remember, both excuses and conscious choices are products of your own mind, a mind that is working exactly the way it is supposed to work. To make sure that you've chosen consciously requires that you are awake long enough to truly look at your choice and compare it to your goals.

For the purpose of staying on your diet, this will only take a second or two at a time, but can be the difference between choosing yogurt with fruit for breakfast instead of a donut, and a salad for lunch instead of French-fries.

But even if you are awake for those few seconds while the menu is in your hands, you still can't choose the right food to attain your goal unless you have an actual goal in mind before you ever sit down at the table. A specific, reachable, quantifiable goal is absolutely essential in order to take control.

This means taking the time to find an eating program that will really help you lose weight and at the same time help you regain your health. Take the time to study that program so that you will be able to tell when you've stepped outside the lines.

As I've suggested earlier in this book, my own recommendation is the book by Dr. Joel Fuhrman, *Eat to Live: The Revolutionary Formula for Fast and Sustained Weight Loss*. This book works with your body, so that you can eat as much as you want and still lose weight. In fact, as Dr. Fuhrman points out, if you're eating the right things, the more you eat the thinner you get. If you continue to feed your body with fruit or vegetables whenever you have a desire for something sweet, you will be using your own cravings to get healthy and thin.

What if you've already eaten the candy bar?

Oh well, we can't win them all. But this is a wonderful opportunity to listen to that excuse you make up for eating something that goes against your dietary goals.

It is far easier to see what happens if we watch someone else doing it for a minute:

Imagine that you have a friend who has every intention of losing weight, who is totally committed, and

who may even have gone to the expense of joining a gym —
but who helped herself to a donut this morning when the
boss brought them in as a treat for the office. She notices
that you notice, and looks a bit sheepish. And then she
says "I didn't have time to have breakfast this morning."

If your friend is a Zen master, or if she regularly
attends Alcoholics Anonymous meetings, she'll notice that
she has just done some "stinking thinking." And, hopefully,
she'll be able to laugh at herself and go on with her day
without beating herself up about it.

The decision to eat the Big Mac® and super-sized
fries was made by the unconscious mind, and that decision
was rationalized by the conscious mind. At the moment
that it was happening, your friend may not have felt as
though she had a lot of choice. She may even have carried
on an internal argument between the self that wants so
badly to meet her weight loss goals, and the excuse that
causes her to slide.

If you're arguing with yourself, you lose. But hey —
somebody has to!

So what happens when you're in this situation, and
you've just eaten the chocolate decadence cheesecake (or
anything else that isn't on your chosen eating plan)?

Use the skills you've learned during walking
meditation, and replace the excuse (whatever it might be),
with an honest statement. Instead of "Just one won't hurt,"
say to yourself, "I'm drinking this Pepsi® because I want to,
even though I know it will make me fat."

In the book *The Four Agreements: A Practical Guide to
Personal Freedom*, by Don Miguel Ruiz, the very first rule is
"Be impeccable with your word." Honesty is a very powerful
force, and internal honesty is just as important as telling
the truth to your friends and family. It eliminates the need
to support excuses for behavior that actually embarrasses
you (doing something that you didn't really want to do) and

lets you use the leftover energy for something else — like living your life.

No, it won't change the fact that you've just eaten something that you promised yourself you wouldn't eat. But it makes the decision a conscious one. In a strange way, you are actually using your mistakes and moments of weakness to reinforce the strength of your conscious mind, becoming awake to what is really happening, and taking conscious responsibility for your own eating choices!

And tomorrow you may surprise yourself when you say, almost without thinking, "No, but thank you very much" to that sweet blob of non-food.

Do you ever lose the desire for sugar, fat and salt?

No, you cannot change human nature.

If you are hoping that someday you will be able to let down your guard and simply eat anything you want, you're dreaming. Our appetites cannot tell the difference between deadly sugar and health-giving fruit (although the body can tell the difference when it's faced with repairing the damage and storing the unwanted calories).

You will also go on wanting fat, in spite of the fact that excess fat in the diet causes heart disease and some kinds of cancer. Your appetites will never change, because they are ruled by your survival system.

But the more you practice walking meditation, and learn to reduce the excess stress in your life, the easier it is to make good eating choices. If you replace your old, unhealthy diet with one filled with plenty of fruits and vegetables, you will eventually find that you can use your desire for sweetness to lead you to food that improves your health and reduces your weight.

Now, there are things you can do to make this process even easier. Because you are totally committed to weight loss and good health, you will want to arrange your

How to Keep Your Commitment

environment so that you have taken away as many obstacles as possible.

Action Step #8

In Action Step #7 we talked about "cheating." I know that you're serious about following the Weight Loss: How to Keep Your Commitment Program, and that means you're washing away all negative, self-destructive thoughts like "cheating,"

But what if this happens:

You walk in to the office snack room with the intention of buying an expensive bottle of water from the pop machine. But your mind is on that project you're working on at your desk. Your fingers are on automatic pilot — and they punch in the code for "Pepsi." Now you're looking at that can of sugar water in your hand (or drinking that can of sugar water).

Have you just started on the slippery path to failure?

No. We're not thinking thoughts like that any more, remember?

You now have a perfect opportunity to analyze what just happened, so you can arrange your day to keep it from happening again. And don't jump to the easy conclusions. You may be surprised by what you learn if you stop to really think about it.

We tend to operate on automatic pilot at specific times. Daydreaming is a necessary activity, when the mind gets to dig down deep into our subconscious in order to tap into our most creative impulses. But daydreaming — or any time when you are concentrating on the images and thoughts inside your head instead of seeing the real world you're standing in — can put your instinctive cravings in charge of your actions.

If your blood sugar is low, or you're stressed out or tired, your subconscious mind will try to lead you to sugar.

When your conscious mind gets the signal that a subconscious decision has been made — often before it's even acted on — you'll hear the automatic excuse (as a thought) that "explains" the decision that your conscious mind can't remember making. I know that's a difficult concept to grasp, but neuroscientists have proven that it happens to all of us.

The problem is, most of us argue with ourselves after a slip in our diets, or put ourselves down. That isn't useful.

Instead, look at the situation closely.

If you have sugar in your hand (or something made with white flour), it may be a signal that your blood sugar is low, or you've become stressed or tired. Did you have refined carbohydrates for breakfast instead of oatmeal or fruit? Did you skip breakfast? Did you drink too much coffee? Have you worked for too long without taking a break? Do you need to get up and move around a little, to get away from the problem you're working on?

If the slip involves fat-filled food, like a hamburger or potato chips, you could be operating out of habit. Fat isn't addictive, but we like the taste — and we love all that extra salt that they always put on high-fat snacks.

And you might notice that the most popular fast-food items, like deluxe hamburgers and pizza, include lots of white flour and even sugar in the bun, crust, and secret sauce. The best way to avoid these obstacles to health is to keep them out of your house, and keep out of the stores that sell them.

Recovering alcoholics are willing to drive home the long way around in order to keep from driving past the bars they used to hang out in. Are you willing to do that, if it would help you stay away from fattening fast food?

Ask yourself these questions: Do these "slips" happen at the same time every day? Do they happen every time you start thinking about a particular problem, or when a specific memory pops into your mind? Do you find yourself eating out of habit when your creativity is engaged in an exciting project?

Once you've spent the time to discover the actual obstacle, it's time to find a way to get around it. What needs to change so that your body will get the nutrition it's calling for? How can you make sure you always have healthy, non-fattening food available when you need it? What action do you need to take, at this specific time, to move you closer to your goals?

There — isn't that much more positive and life-affirming than picking on yourself because you made a mistake?

If you practice this often enough, you will be able to go through the process, and correct your course, before the slip is acted on. When that starts happening, you know that you're on the road to success — just watch as the pounds melt off, and your health improves.

Practical stuff #1:
Get your house in order.

Seven years ago, when I started searching for a way to bring myself out of mild, chronic depression and to put more control back in my life, I came to the conclusion that one of the first things I should do is look at the part of the environment that I could easily control — my own home.

I began to pay very close attention to the way I felt when people came into my house. If I usually became anxious, disturbed, or angry when certain people came to visit, they simply didn't get invited any more. I became committed to turning my home into a sanctuary, where I could feel truly safe from emotional distress.

When people kick their addictions to drugs or alcohol they understand that their success will depend upon keeping these dangerous substances out of their homes. They may even need to change the places where they spend their time, and choose new friends who can have fun without using drugs or drinking. You have just started on a program that will break your addiction to sugar and fat, and you will need to be just as diligent about keeping your environment safe as any other recovering addict.

To make my home safe for my new healthy diet, the first thing I did was clean out my cupboards. I love to bake bread, cookies and (especially) cinnamon rolls, and had been steadily gaining weight because of all the wonderful new recipes I was trying. I knew if the ingredients were in the house, it would be hard to keep myself from baking. So I threw away all the white flour, yeast and sugar in my house.

I know someone who is committed to keeping her diet sugar-free, but who loves to bake. She continues to create wonderful baked goods each weekend when she has the time to pursue this hobby, and then gives the cakes, cookies and bread to her friends.

If she truly understood how dangerous these substances are to the human body, I know she would get rid of all those unhealthy ingredients and take up a different creative activity. If it isn't good for your body, it isn't good for your friends and family, either.

I cannot stress how much easier it is to keep your commitment to weight loss if you get rid your home of all unhealthy food.

Clearly, since you tend to eat more (and gain more weight) when there is more unhealthy food in the house, it makes sense to get rid of everything in your cupboards that you know you shouldn't be eating.

If you eat a piece of toast in the morning made with white bread, and your chosen diet encourages whole grains, the reasonable thing to do is get rid of the white bread in your house. Then throw away the butter in the fridge and replace it with unsweetened apple butter or other non-fat, non-sugared topping. Look at your chosen weight-loss plan carefully, and create an environment in which it can work.

This step looks easy, but everyone fights it. We hate waste, and we remember all those starving kids in North Korea. It seems criminal to throw away good food. But

Weight Loss:

remember — it isn't good food if it makes you fat, clogs up your arteries, leads to diabetes and heart disease, or causes cancer. Remember — mice like the taste of D-Con.

But what if your family or roommates don't want to join you in your diet? Then compromise is going to be needed. Some part of the kitchen will need to be set aside as yours, and yours alone.

Make it clear that you can't eat those cookies in your husband's cupboard because they don't belong to you. This will become easier as you continue to practice walking meditation, and become more comfortable with making conscious eating choices. But it will definitely be easier to make those conscious choices if the environment you live in is safe.

Of course, you can't know if a given food is one you should keep, or one you should throw away, if you haven't chosen a specific diet program. If you breezed right through the chapter on choosing a diet, go back and do this step now. Remember — responsible choices are made when we consider the natural outcomes of a given choice, and compare it to our intended goal. Having that goal is absolutely essential if you are to begin making healthy choices.

Next, go through the menus that you have created, or which are provided in your diet book, and make sure your cupboards are stocked with the ingredients you'll need. Make your weight loss plan easy to carry out by being prepared. Enthusiasm is a lot easier to maintain if you aren't constantly running to the store for an unusual ingredient that your new recipes call for.

The process of planning is actually the first step towards becoming more conscious and aware of the choices you make.

By planning your program and creating a safe place in which to carry it out, you are taking conscious control. And that's the true secret of success.

If you have children in the house this step is absolutely crucial. The number of overweight children in America is astounding. While the invention of computer games and TV may be part of the problem, it is incredibly important to make sure that their young bodies are being built with the healthiest food available.

A child who is overweight may have a weight problem for the rest of her life. While you cannot control the choices your children make in the lunchroom cafeteria, the available foods at home should always be healthy.

Practical stuff #2:
Check your progress.

I had to do some serious thinking recently, after I brought food into my house that I don't normally choose to eat, "because I had company coming and wanted to have something here that they would enjoy."

OK, you recognize the "stinking thinking" in that last paragraph. Healthy food is just as enjoyable as unhealthy food, but I lapsed. It happens. And I know it isn't possible to gain five pounds from a loaf of bread, some butter, and some ham in three days time. But I did. (*The False Fat Diet* by Elson M. Haas, M.D. may explain some of the reasons why.)

Fortunately, I had been weighing myself on a regular basis, and was able to catch myself before I had regained all the weight that I had worked so hard to lose.

Remember, human nature doesn't change, so it is easy to slip back into old habits and eat the foods that are not conducive to good heath. You will want to check up on your progress on a regular basis, and continue to do so long after you have achieved your ideal weight. We all lapse, but if we let down our guard, a small five-pound gain can become 30 or 50 pounds all too quickly.

Checking the scales is the most obvious way to do this. The way your clothes feel is also useful, but it's easier to catch a few extra pounds by watching your scale. If you find you've been moving back up in weight, go back to the skills you know you already have, be totally honest with yourself about changes you have recently made that are sabotaging your success, and you will soon be back on track.

Practical stuff #3:
Get the support you need.

Several chapters ago you learned a simple meditation that will allow you to feel loved any time you need the extra spiritual hug. You're starting on a new journey in life, and you can use all the hugs you can get.

During this process, one of the best forms of support you can give yourself is knowledge. Commit yourself to getting a deep understanding of the way the body works, and what you really need to eat in order to lose weight and support your health. One of the best ways to do this is to read the book by Dr. Fuhrman that I've recommended so many times in this book.

But what about getting support from your family — your spouse and children, and possibly even parents? What about getting some needed support from your coworkers and friends?

You have a right to ask for this support. In fact, you have a right to ask for anything that you need or want. But don't expect it. If you do, you may be disappointed. And you might use that disappointment as an excuse to give up your goals of losing weight and getting healthy.

Actually, when you think about it, since it is you that is changing, it is actually your family members and friends who will be most in need of support. Someone that they love is changing, becoming more self-sufficient — different. And that is sometimes a very scary thing.

It can be especially scary for other people in your life if you're meeting your weight-loss goals by becoming stronger and more self-aware. This, of course, is what this book is trying to teach you to do.

For that reason, it is extremely important that you build weight-loss goals that do not require huge commitments from your friends and family. Share your goals with them, certainly. But always remember that this is something that you are doing for yourself.

It is your body you see in the mirror each day. It is your clothes that no longer fit. It is your arteries that are getting clogged with fat and cholesterol. You are the one who has a higher risk of heart disease, diabetes and cancer.

Changing that body and becoming healthier is something that only you can do. If you find yourself needing your family and friends to do something different than they are doing now, you are setting yourself up for failure.

But let's face it — changing other people is a full-time job for many of us. I personally spent 48 years on that job, before I put myself on this program and became aware of what I was doing. When I finally "woke up" I realized that I had been perpetually angry and disappointed by all the things that I believed other people were doing wrong, or for things I didn't get because other people didn't give them to me. This is a classic symptom of what is now commonly called co-dependency.

If you live under chronic, self-induced stress, the negative thoughts that you carry around with you may often be pictures of arguments or disappointments that happen because someone hasn't done or been what you thought you needed.

Now that you are totally committed to your weight-loss goals, you cannot afford to create that kind of negativity. Since the best way to create disappointment with a loved one is to expect something that they don't want to give you, the best way to avoid that disappointment is to ask for that support, but to not need it if it isn't offered. Let them love you their way.

But what if their way is to bring home cakes, cookies, high-fat roasts and other "goodies" that you would have loved last week, but which you're committed to avoid now?

You will be at an advantage if you are the one in the household who gets to do the shopping and cooking. If you find a great cookbook with enticing, healthy recipes, you can create a meal that the whole family will enjoy without ever having to tell them that it's helping you lose weight.

If there's a cake sitting on the counter when you're finished with your meal, ask to be excused while the rest of the family enjoys it. Please don't waste your precious energy telling them that the sugar and white flour in the cake isn't good for them.

Put the cake away in a cupboard or the fridge when everyone is done, and make sure that you have a fascinating project to go to when the dishes are cleaned up and put away. You'll forget the cake is there if you have something else that truly occupies your mind.

If the family has been bringing home sweets as treats for you for many years, they may continue for a while just because they still aren't sure that you're committed. Give them a break — they're trying to be nice. If the sweets really are for you, and you gently ignore them for a while, your family will stop buying them. But give them ideas for other treats that you might like, such as flowers or books, so they still have that opportunity to show that they love you.

Another way that they can show their love for you, if they choose to become involved in your weight-loss project at all, is to go with you to the library or bookstore and help you pick out a cookbook that has healthy recipes with mouth-watering pictures of food that everyone would enjoy.

But if they show no interest in your desire to lose weight — don't sweat it. This is your fight, not theirs. If you make sure to remain supportive of their needs while also becoming more supportive of your own, they will eventually realize that your new-found enthusiasm for health is not going to hurt them or their relationship with you.

Whom do you turn to for support?

The best people to count on for support when you're on a diet are people who have the same commitment that you do.

The book *The Town That Lost a Ton* tells about three women who created a support group that came to include hundreds of people. If you're an organizing sort of person, the book will give you some great examples of exactly how to put something like that together, along with weekly projects and handouts for your group.

The Weight Watchers™ and Jenny Craig™ programs have also been very successful in creating this kind of supportive atmosphere, although they aren't free. The appeal to this type of program is the structure that comes from specified meal plans and group support. If it appeals for you, you can find your local chapter online.

Because these programs concentrate on giving smaller portions of the "average" American diet, they are not as healthy as eating the diet found in the diet program designed by Dr. Joel Fuhrman. For that reason, I don't personally recommend them, but many people have used them successfully to lose weight.

You might also get some of the support you need from the local health club, which probably has classes where you can meet other people who are in the same stage of their own weight-loss programs, and who would love to have a new friend. Your community college or parks department might also have classes that would allow you to meet like-minded people.

If you are having a hard time keeping your commitment to exercise regularly, but don't want to join a gym — and you don't know anyone else who is interested in doing anything with you — check out my daughter's website at http://WomensExerciseNetwork.com. She provides a free forum where you can find other people interested in the same activities, and who are at the same fitness level.

As Jessie says on her site, "Don't get discouraged if your friends don't want to run, bike, hike or swim with you — just find new friends!" Of course, you'll want to use some common sense while arranging to meet someone you don't know.

And don't forget that sometimes the most supportive activities have absolutely nothing to do with food or losing weight!

If you have been wanting to learn how to paint for years, but just never got around to it, go ahead and sign up for a night class now. It will give you something exciting to do on those evenings that you might otherwise have spent in front of the TV, eating chips. You'll meet new people, and your friendships with them are unlikely to revolve around food.

Or you might find that it isn't people that you need, as much as a project. Did you once love building intricate model airplanes or cars, but somehow lost interest? Maybe now is the time to take it up again.

Take a real long look at what you really enjoy doing. This isn't as easy as you would expect, because many of us give up the things we enjoy when family and work responsibilities increase. You might have the time to do them now, but you may have forgotten how important they used to be.

For that reason, it really might take a full weekend, or even longer, to rediscover the talent you once used or the activity you once enjoyed. You might even find something completely new, an interest that engages your mind and that could involve you in an exciting new project.

Have you ever been so engrossed in a project or hobby that you forgot to eat? That's exactly what you need right now. It will make a big difference in the quality of your life, and can really help you lose weight.

You're on your way!

You now have everything you need to stay committed to your weight-loss goals. If you haven't already done so, find a book that outlines a nutritional program that you feel comfortable with, and which fits your needs and lifestyle. Remember — don't just pick the program that worked for your neighbor or coworkers. We all have different bodies and needs.

As I have already mentioned (can you tell how important I think it is)? I suggest the book *Eat to Live: The Revolutionary Formula for Fast and Sustained Weight Loss* by Dr. Joel Fuhrman. It gives you a thorough understanding of the reasons why you need to give yourself the fruits and vegetables your body craves. This is the diet I used myself to lose 37 pounds in four months, so I know it works.

Remember to practice the walking meditation that you learned at the beginning of the book, and occasionally practice the meditation that teaches you what it feels like to love yourself. These simple mental exercises will help you "wake up" and make fully conscious decisions about your diet and your health.

If you do discover that your instinctual mind has made an eating choice for you, use that experience to practice total honesty, and let it reinforce your ability to accept full responsibility for your choices. You can use your mistakes as stepping-stones on the way to full freedom from instinctual cravings.

Since the instinctual mind is more apt to gain control and make your eating choices for you if you live in chronic stress, promise yourself that you will do whatever it takes to remove the excess stress from your life. Your success (and happiness) depend on it.

Remember to use memories of past successes, at anything, as a blueprint for success with your weight-loss plan.

Remember to laugh, even at yourself, and to find projects or activities that are enjoyable and fascinating. Now is the time when you should live life to the fullest. Have fun!

You are on your way to becoming thinner, healthier, and more energetic. As you continue to practice walking meditation you may find yourself meeting many other goals that are completely unconnected to weight loss, simply because you're more focused and awake. These are just some of the wonderful side effects of your commitment to good health!

A personal note from the author:

My life has changed so much since I kicked the habits that made me fat — and I really have become a crusader. Every day I see the huge personal and social costs of obesity.

Because I really care about your health, I hope you will take a few moments to write to me about your experiences with this book. Let me know if it has helped, and how — or tell me how you think I could improve it. Your opinion is important to me. If you would let me use your comments in my newsletter or on my website, please let me know. Just send an e-mail to me directly at jonni@howtothinkthin.com. I value your input, and hope to hear from you soon.

Yours in good health,

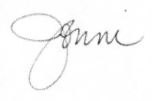

Suggested reading

This is a list of some of my favorite books on the human mind, meditation, and change. I'm an obsessive reader, but to keep this short, I've only included a few of the books I've read and loved. Enjoy.

The Undiscovered Mind: How the Human Brain Defies Replication, Medication, and Explanation
by John Horgan

Many interesting studies are discussed that shows how the mind works — and how much we still don't know about our own brains.

Psycho-Pictography: The New Way to Use the Miracle Power of Your Mind
by Vernon Howard

This is a wonderfully engaging book that shows how to use mental images to regain conscious awareness and institute change. I have given away at least five copies of this one, because it's one of my favorite books. It is now unavailable, but you can easily find used ones, and it's well worth the effort.

Heart of the Mind: Engaging Your Inner Power to Change With Neuro-Linguistic Programming
by Connirae Andreas, Steve Andreas

This book gives you a "front-row seat" in following the accounts of people whose lives have been changed and whose dreams became reality by using their own inner power to change with NLP. The authors include a step-by-step understanding of how each change occurred, that you can use for those areas in your life that you want to be different.

The Zen of Eating: Ancient Answers to Modern Weight Problems
by Ronna Kabatznick

From a Buddhist perspective, overeating is a disorder of desire. This book will teach readers how to find freedom from eating problems and the tyranny of desire that triggers them. Filled with concrete, practical exercises and the wisdom of the ages.

The Four Agreements: A Practical Guide to Personal Freedom
by Don Miguel Ruiz

I once had the pleasure of hearing Don Miguel Ruiz speak, and he is absolutely mesmerizing. His speaking style carries over very well in this powerful little book. It is written in a simple, yet sophisticated style, and makes these ancient ideas about personal strength through conscious awareness easy to understand and put into practice.

The Seduction of Madness: Revolutionary Insights into the World of Psychosis and a Compassionate Approach to Recovery at Home
by Edward M. Podvoll

This book is out of print, but it looks like it is now available from Amazon.com, and I've ordered myself another copy. The book is written by an amazingly compassionate man who practices a form of psychiatry that incorporates the philosophy of Tibetan Buddhists and the Lakota Sioux. You will never read another book like it.

Crazy   *Wisdom*
by Chogyam Trungpa, Sherab Chodzin

I first discovered walking meditation, the basis for all the mental exercises in this book, by reading a book by Chogyam Trungpa. That original book is no longer in print, but this one promises to bring you much more deeply into the ways of Tibetan Buddhism, in a way that is applicable to the modern Western lifestyle.

One Bowl: A Guide to Eating for Body and Spirit
by Don Gerrard

This book proposes a simple but extraordinarily powerful idea: By adopting a single bowl as the vessel for your meals, you will become more aware of the food you eat, how you eat, and the effects (large and small) of particular foods on your body and your spiritual and physical well-being.

112

LaVergne, TN USA
29 November 2009
165478LV00006B/38/A